CPR AND AED

National Safety Council

CAll 911 FIRST
AED USED 3 TIME IN A ROW →
AND ANALISE PACIENT - PERSON

McGraw Hill Higher Education

Boston Burr Ridge, IL Dubuque, IA Madison, WI New York
San Francisco St. Louis Bangkok Bogotá Caracas Kuala Lumpur
Lisbon London Madrid Mexico City Milan Montreal New Delhi
Santiago Seoul Singapore Sydney Taipei Toronto

The McGraw·Hill Companies

Higher Education

CPR AND AED

Published by McGraw-Hill, a business unit of The McGraw-Hill Companies, Inc., 1221 Avenue of the Americas, New York, NY 10020.
Some ancillaries, including electronic and print components, may not be available to customers outside the United States.

This book is printed on acid-free paper.

4 5 6 7 8 9 0 QWD/QWD 0 9 8 7 6 5

ISBN 0–07–301676–4

Publisher: *David T. Culverwell*
Senior Sponsoring Editor: *Roxan Kinsey*
Developmental Editor: *Patricia Forrest*
Editorial Coordinator: *Connie Kuhl*
Outside Managing Editor: *Kelly Trakalo*
Outside Production Editor: *Marilyn Rothenberger*
Marketing Manager: *Lynn M. Kalb*
Senior Project Manager: *Sheila M. Frank*
Senior Production Supervisor: *Laura Fuller*
Lead Media Project Manager: *Audrey A. Reiter*
Media Technology Producer: *Janna Martin*
Senior Coordinator of Freelance Design: *Michelle D. Whitaker*
Cover/Interior Designer: *Seann Dwyer/Studio Montage, St. Louis, MO*
Lead Photo Research Coordinator: *Carrie K. Burger*
Photo Research: *Karen Pugliano*
Supplement Producer: *Brenda A. Ernzen*
Compositor and Art Studio: *Electronic Publishing Services Inc., NYC*
Typeface: *11.5/13 Minion*
Printer: *Quebecor World Dubuque*

All photos © The McGraw-Hill Companies, Inc./Rick Brady, photographer

Illustrations by Electronic Publishing Services Inc.: Jennifer Brumbaugh–3.1, 4.6;
Matthew McAdams–1.1, 4.1, 4.4, 5.1, 5.2, 5.5.

The information presented in this book is based on the current recommendations of responsible medical and industrial sources at the time of printing. The National Safety Council and the publisher, however, make no guarantee as to, and assume no responsibility for, correctness, sufficiency or completeness of such information or recommendations. Other or additional safety measures may be required under particular circumstances.

www.mhhe.com

About the National Safety Council

Founded in 1913, the National Safety Council (NSC) is a nonprofit membership organization devoted to protecting life and promoting health. Its mission "is to educate and influence society to adopt safety, health, and environmental policies, practices, and procedures that prevent and mitigate, human suffering and economic losses arising from preventable causes."

The National Safety Council has been the leader in protecting life and promoting health in the workplace for over 90 years. The Council has helped make great improvements in workplace safety, and expanded their focus to include safety on the roads and in the home and community. Working through its 37,000 members, and in partnership with public agencies, private groups, and other associations, the Council serves as an impartial information gathering and distribution organization; it disseminates safety, health, and environmental materials from its Itasca, Illinois, headquarters through a network of regional offices, chapters, and training centers.

In 1990 NSC established First Aid and CPR courses to promote effective emergency response. Since then, they have grown to meet the changing needs of emergency responders at all levels of expertise. Upon successful completion of this course, you join more than 10 million National Safety Council trained responders protecting life and promoting health.

Acknowledgements

The National Safety Council wishes to thank the following Chapters and individuals for their assistance in developing this program:

For providing technical advice and assistance with photography: Safety Council of Maryland and Ms. Pat Raven, Director, Occupational Services, Safety Council of Maryland.

For providing technical advice and assistance with videotaping: the Arizona Chapter, National Safety Council, John Stubbs and C. J. Anderson.

For providing technical writing services: Tom Lochhaas, Editorial Services, Newburyport, MA.

For providing direction and support for National Safety Council Emergency Care programs: Donna M. Siegfried, Executive Director, Emergency Care & Home and Community Programs; Barbara Caracci, Director of Emergency Care Products and Training; Donna Fredenhagen, Manager of National Programs and Initiatives; Kathy Safranek, Project Administrator.

Publisher's Acknowledgements

Jason J. Goetz
Senior Safety Engineer
Worldwide Environmental, Health & Safety
Intel Corporation
Phoenix, AZ

James H. Howson
Director, Emergency Preparedness
New Jersey Hospital
Princeton, NJ

Debbie Kaye
Instructor, Dakota County Technical College
Minnesota Safety Council
Rosemont, MN

Tom Link
Safety and Health Council of North Carolina
Harrisburg, NC

Robb Rehberg, Ph.D.
Director and Chief, Emergency Medical Services
Montclair State University
Upper Montclair, NJ

Lisa Webb
Coordinator, Business Continuity & Disaster Recovery Planning
Delta Airlines

B. Drew Wellmon, D.O.
Wellmon Family Practice
Shippenburg, PA

Table of Contents

Chapter

1 Take Action in an Emergency

CHAPTER PREVIEW

- The Emergency Medical Services System
- Legal Considerations
- Taking Action in an Emergency
- Avoiding Infectious Diseases

Cardiopulmonary resuscitation (CPR) and use of an automated external defibrillator (AED) are two of the most important first aid skills because they can help save lives. With this manual you will learn how to perform these skills, along with related skills such as rescue breathing and care for a choking victim. All of these skills together are called basic life support (BLS). When a victim's breathing or heart stops, no matter what the reason or cause, you can use these valuable skills to help keep the victim alive until advanced medical care is available.

The Emergency Medical Services System

Workers and citizens who are trained in first aid are the first step in the Emergency Medical Services (EMS) system. As a first aider you are *only* the first step, so part of your responsibility is to make sure the Emergency Medical Services system responds to help a victim of injury or sudden illness by calling 911 (or your local or company emergency number). You will learn more about calling EMS later in this chapter. In most communities in the United States, help will arrive within minutes. The first aid you give helps the victim until then.

Legal Considerations

Can You Be Sued for Giving First Aid?

Generally you do not need to be concerned about being sued for performing CPR or giving other first aid. If you give first aid as you are trained in this course, and do your best, there is little chance of being found legally liable. To protect yourself, follow these guidelines:

1. Act *only* as you are trained to act.
2. Get a victim's consent before giving first aid.
3. Do not move a victim unnecessarily.
4. Call for professional help.
5. Keep giving care until help arrives.

Good Samaritan Laws

Most states have laws called **Good Samaritan laws** designed to encourage people to help others in an emergency without worrying about being sued. These laws protect you legally when you give first aid. It is unlikely you would be found liable or financially responsible for a victim's injury as long as you follow the guidelines mentioned above. Ask your instructor about the specific Good Samaritan laws in your area.

Must You Give First Aid?

In most states you have no legal obligation to give first aid as a citizen or a bystander at the scene of an emergency. As the specific obligations may vary, ask your instructor about the law in your area. If you do begin giving first aid, however, you are obligated to continue giving care if you can and to remain with the victim.

Your job may require giving first aid, and that does make you legally obligated. This is called a **duty to act.** Off the job, however, depending on your state's laws, you are usually not legally required to give first aid except in special cases, such as parents or guardians caring for their child and other special situations.

Get the Victim's Consent

A responsive (awake and alert) victim must give consent before you can give first aid. Tell the person you have been trained and describe what you will do to help. The person may give consent by telling you it is okay or by nodding agreement.

An unresponsive victim, however, is assumed to give consent for your help—this is called **implied consent.** Similarly, consent is assumed if a parent or guardian is not present and a child needs first aid.

Follow Standards of Care

Legally, you may be liable for the results of your actions if you do not follow accepted standards of care. **Standard of care** refers to what others with your same training would do in a similar situation. It is important you do only as you are trained. Any other actions could result in the injury or illness becoming worse.

You may be guilty of **negligence** if:

1. You have a duty to act.
2. You breach that duty (by not acting or acting incorrectly).
3. Your actions or inaction causes injury or damages (including such things as physical injury or pain).

Examples of negligent actions could include moving a victim unnecessarily, doing something you have not been trained to do, or failing to give first aid as you have been trained.

Once you begin giving CPR or other first aid, do not stop until another trained person takes over. Stay with the victim until help arrives or someone with equal or greater training takes over. If you leave the victim and the injury or illness becomes worse, this is called **abandonment.** Note that abandonment is different from justified instances of stopping care, such as if you are exhausted and unable to continue or you are in imminent danger because of hazards at the scene.

Taking Action in an Emergency

Follow these steps in any emergency:

1. Recognize the emergency and check the scene.
2. Decide to help.
3. Call 911.
4. Check the victim.
5. Give first aid.

Recognize the Emergency and Check the Scene

You usually know there is an emergency when you see one. You may see an unresponsive person lying on the ground, an injured or ill victim, or someone acting strangely.

Always check the scene when you recognize an emergency has occurred—before rushing in to help a victim. You must be safe yourself if you are to help another. Look for any hazards such as the following:

- Smoke, flames
- Spilled chemicals, vapors
- Downed electrical wires
- Risk of explosion, building collapse
- Roadside dangers, high-speed traffic
- Potential personal violence

If the scene is dangerous, ***stay away and call for help.*** Do not become a victim yourself!

As part of checking the scene, look to see if there are other victims. More help may be needed for multiple victims. Look also for any clues that may help you determine what happened and what first aid may be needed. As well, look for bystanders who may be able to help give first aid or go to a telephone to call 911.

Learning Checkpoint 1

1. True or False: Good Samaritan laws protect only professionals like paramedics and health-care providers.

2. True or False: The best thing to do in any emergency is move the victim to your car and get to an emergency room.

3. You have a duty to act when:

   a. You stop at the scene of an emergency

   b. You have taken a first aid course

   c. You have a first aid kit with you

   d. Your job requires you to give first aid when needed

4. Check off which victims you have consent to give first aid to:

   _____ a. An unresponsive victim

   _____ b. A child without parent or guardian present

   _____ c. All victims, all of the time

   _____ d. A victim who nods when you ask if it is okay to give first aid

   _____ e. A child whose parent or guardian gives consent for the child

5. Check off things you should always do when giving first aid:

   _____ a. Move the victim

   _____ b. Do what you have been trained to do

   _____ c. Try any first aid technique you have read or heard about

   _____ d. Ask for victim's consent

   _____ e. Stay with the victim until another trained person takes over

   _____ f. Transport all victims to the emergency room in your vehicle

Decide to Help

When you see a victim and the scene is safe, you need to decide to help that victim. This is not always easy. You may be worried about not doing the right thing but remember that you have first aid training. Once you call for help, professionals will be there very soon. Your goal is to help the victim until they take over. Do not delay giving first aid because you hope someone else will do it—realize that it is up to you.

Call 911

Call 911 (or your local or company emergency number) immediately if you recognize a life-threatening injury or illness. A life-threatening emergency is one in which a problem threatens the victim's airway, breathing, or circulation of blood, as described in Chapter 2. Do not try to transport a victim to the emergency room yourself in such cases. Movement may worsen the victim's condition, or the victim may suddenly need additional care on the way. If you are not sure whether a situation is serious enough to call, do not hesitate—call 911. It is better to be safe than sorry.

If the victim is responsive and may not be seriously injured or ill, go on to the next step to check the victim before calling 911—and then call 911 or a healthcare provider if needed.

Always call 911 when:

- The victim may have a life-threatening condition
- The victim is unresponsive
- The victim's condition may become life threatening
- Moving the victim could make his or her condition worse

A victim may say his or her condition is not all that serious. For example, heart attack victims often say they just have "indigestion" even when they have other heart attack signs and symptoms. You should call 911 anyway and let the dispatch center decide if the situation is an emergency.

In addition to calling 911 for injury or illness, call in these situations:

- Fire, explosion
- Vehicle crash
- Downed electrical wire
- Chemical spill, gas leak, or the presence of any unknown substances

How to Call EMS

When you call 911 or your local emergency number, be ready to give the following information:

- Your name and the phone number you are using
- The location and number of victims—specific enough for the arriving crew to find them
- What happened to the victim(s) and any special circumstances or conditions that may require special rescue or medical equipment
- The victim's condition: For example, is the victim responsive? Breathing? Bleeding?
- The victim's approximate age and sex
- What is being done for the victim(s)

Do not hang up until the dispatcher instructs you to, as you may be given advice on how to care for the victim.

If another responsible person is present, ask him or her to call 911 while you go on to check the victim and give needed care (**Figure 1-1**).

Check the Victim

Check the victim for life-threatening conditions requiring immediate first aid (see Chapter 2).

Give First Aid

Give first aid once you have checked the victim and know his or her condition. Note that first aiders do not give medications, even aspirin, to victims because of the risks of allergy or other complications. First aiders can, however, allow adult victims to take medications when appropriate, and in some cases first aiders may assist victims in taking their medications if needed.

Avoiding Infectious Disease

In any emergency situation there is some risk of a first aider getting an infectious disease from a victim who has a disease. That risk is very low, however, and taking steps to prevent being infected greatly reduces that risk.

Bloodborne Disease

Several serious diseases can be transmitted from one person to another through contact with the infected person's blood. These are called **bloodborne**

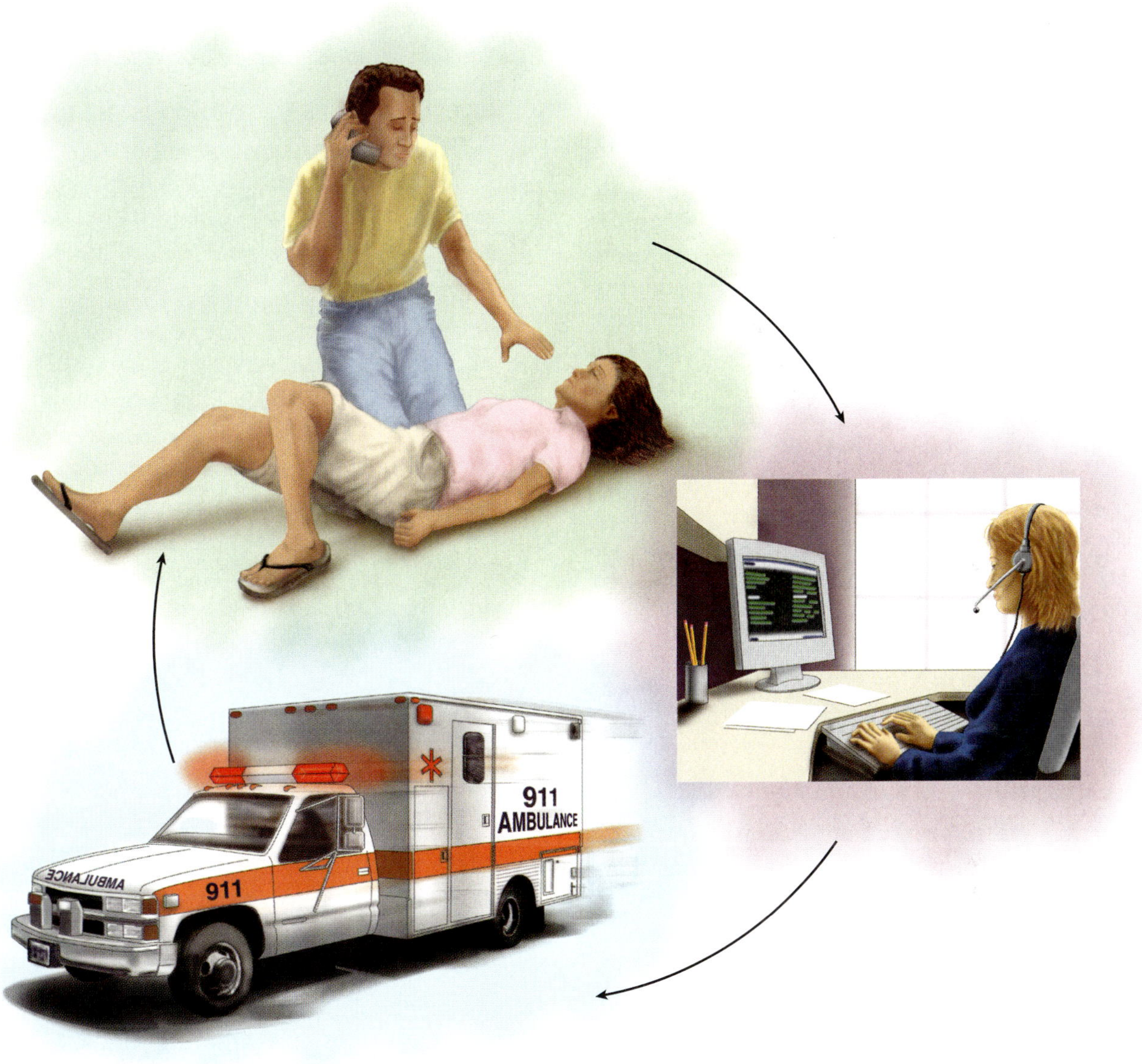

Figure 1-1 Call 911.

diseases. Bacteria or viruses that cause such diseases, called **pathogens,** are also present in some other body fluids, such as semen, vaginal secretions, and bloody saliva or vomit. Other body fluids such as nasal secretions, sweat, tears, and urine do not normally transmit pathogens. Three serious bloodborne infections are HIV, hepatitis B, and hepatitis C.

HIV

The human immunodeficiency virus (HIV) is the pathogen that eventually causes AIDS (acquired immunodeficiency syndrome). AIDS is a fatal disease transmitted from one person to another only through body fluids.

Learning Checkpoint 2

1. True or False: If you see victims injured in an emergency, the first thing to do is get to them quickly and check their condition.

2. When you encounter an injured victim, you should:

a. Give first aid until help arrives

b. Help a victim only if the scene is safe

c. Call 911 for life-threatening injuries

d. All of the above

3. Call 911 for:

a. Medical problems only

b. Police and fire services only

c. Medical problems and fires only

d. Medical problems and all emergencies

Hepatitis B

Hepatitis B (HBV) is a viral infectious disease of the liver also transmitted through contact with an infected person's body fluids. The disease is difficult to treat and often remains in the person for life, possibly leading to liver damage or cancer.

A vaccine is available for HBV. Individuals who are more likely to come in contact with HBV-infected people, such as healthcare workers and professional rescuers, often get this vaccine. The law requires that employees who are at risk for HBV be offered free vaccinations by their employer.

Hepatitis C

Hepatitis C (HCV) is another viral disease that can cause liver disease or cancer. It cannot be cured, and there is no vaccine.

Protection Against Bloodborne Disease

Because bloodborne diseases cannot be cured, they should be prevented. The best prevention is to avoid contact with *all* victims' blood and body fluids. You cannot know whether a victim (even a close friend) is infected, as often these diseases do not produce signs and symptoms. Even victims may not know that they are infected.

WEST NILE VIRUS

West Nile Virus (WNV) is a relatively new bloodborne disease now established as a seasonal epidemic in parts of North America. Less than 1% of people infected with WNV develop severe illness, however, and about 80% have no signs and symptoms at all. WNV is spread mostly by the bite of infected mosquitoes. The best way to avoid WNV is to prevent mosquito bites with personal protection such as wearing long sleeves and pants and reducing mosquito breeding sites.

The Centers for Disease Control and Prevention (CDC) therefore recommends taking **universal precautions** whenever giving first aid. *Universal* means for all victims, all the time, and always assuming that blood and other body fluids may be infected. Use the following recommended precautions to prevent coming into contact with a victim's blood or body fluids:

- Use personal protective equipment (see below)
- If you do not have medical exam gloves with you, put your hands in plastic bags or have the victim dress his or her own wound
- Wash your hands with soap and water before and after giving first aid
- Keep a barrier (gloves or dry cloth) between body fluids and yourself
- Cover any cuts or scrapes in your skin with protective clothing or gloves
- Do not touch your mouth, nose, or eyes when giving first aid (e.g., do not eat, drink, or smoke)
- Do not touch objects soiled with blood or body fluids
- Be careful to avoid being cut by anything sharp at the emergency scene, such as broken glass or torn metal
- Use absorbent material to soak up spilled blood or body fluids, and dispose of it appropriately. Clean the area with a commercial disinfectant or a freshly made 10% bleach solution.
- If you are exposed to a victim's blood or body fluid, wash immediately with soap and water and call your healthcare provider. At work, report the situation to your supervisor.

OSHA requires use of universal precautions by employees who give first aid as part of their job.

Personal Protective Equipment

Personal protective equipment (PPE) is any equipment used to protect yourself from contact with blood or other body fluids. Most important, keep **medical exam gloves** in your first aid kit and wear them in most first aid situations (**Figure 1-2**).

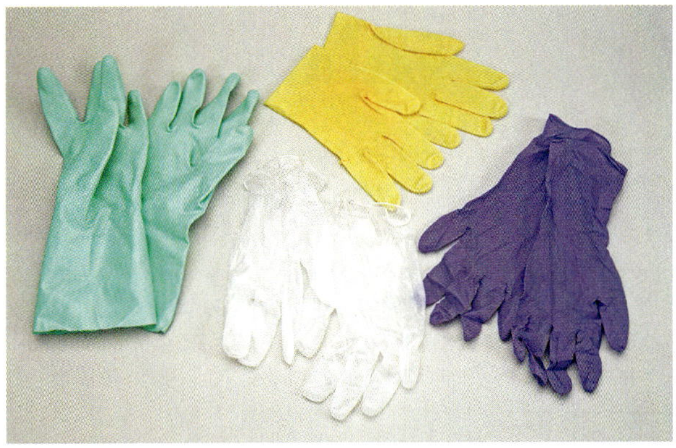

Figure 1-2 Wear gloves to protect yourself from contact with blood or other body fluids.

A pocket face mask or face shield is a barrier device used when giving rescue breathing or CPR. This device should be in the first aid kit, and you should always use it for added protection. Because giving rescue breathing with a barrier device can greatly reduce the chance of an infectious disease being transmitted from or to a victim, barrier devices are recommended (**Figure 1-3**).

Other PPE devices include **eye protection, masks,** and **gowns or aprons.** These are not required in most first aid situations, although OSHA requires such protections be available in some workplaces. In such cases OSHA requires employees to be trained in the use of this PPE. Healthcare workers, for example, are required to wear masks and protective eyewear or face shields during procedures likely to generate droplets of blood or body fluids, and gowns or aprons when blood or body fluid may be splashed. These are called **standard precautions.**

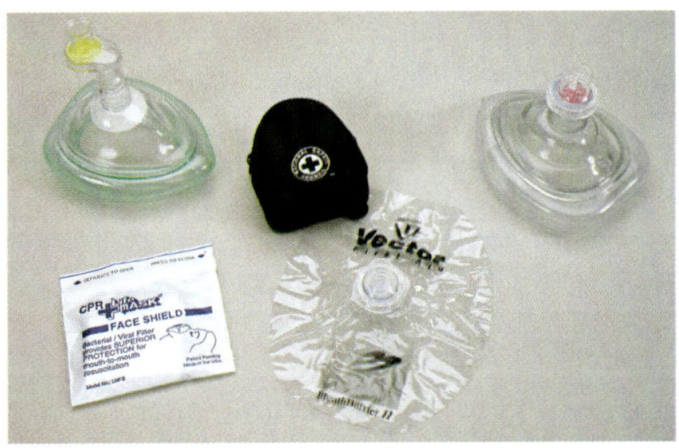

Figure 1-3 Variety of barrier devices.

ALERT

Latex Gloves

Medical exam gloves are often made of latex rubber, to which some people are allergic. Signs and symptoms of latex allergy may include skin rashes, hives, itching eyes or skin, flushing, watery or swollen eyes, runny nose, or an asthmatic reaction. Use gloves made of vinyl or other material if you have any of these symptoms.

Airborne Disease

Infectious diseases may also be transmitted through the air, especially from a victim who is coughing or sneezing. Tuberculosis (TB) has made a comeback in recent decades and is sometimes resistant to treatment.

Healthcare workers sometimes use precautions when caring for people known or suspected to have TB, but rarely does a first aider need to take special precautions against airborne disease.

SARS

In 2003 an outbreak of severe acute respiratory syndrome (SARS) in some parts of the world caused a new scare. SARS is primarily an airborne infectious disease, transmitted when an infected person coughs or sneezes within close proximity of others. During the 2003 epidemic almost 10% of the approximately 8000 known SARS victims in the world died. Only 7 people in the U.S. were known to have contracted SARS, however, all during international travel to epidemic areas. The CDC continues to monitor the risks of SARS and will issue updates and warnings if new outbreaks occur.

First aiders who need or want to learn more about preventing bloodborne and airborne disease are encouraged to take the National Safety Council course on Bloodborne and Airborne Pathogens (www.nsc.org).

Learning Checkpoint 3

1. True or False: Bloodborne diseases are transmitted only through contact with an infected person's blood.

2. True or False: The risk of getting a serious infectious disease by giving first aid is greatly reduced when you take precautions.

3. "Universal precautions" means:

a. Treat all victims as if their body fluids were infected

b. Always wear gloves if blood may be present

c. Do not touch your mouth, nose, or eyes when giving first aid

d. All of the above

4. Check off which of the following situations could lead to getting an infectious disease:

_____ **a.** Touching a bloody bandage in a trash can

_____ **b.** Shaking hands with a person with HIV

_____ **c.** Receiving a hepatitis B vaccination

_____ **d.** Not wearing gloves when providing first aid

_____ **e.** Being near a person with hepatitis C who is coughing

_____ **f.** Contact with an unresponsive victim

Chapter

2 Assess the Victim

CHAPTER PREVIEW

- Check the ABCs
- Get the Victim's History
- Examine the Victim
- Monitor the Victim

After you recognize the emergency, check the scene for safety, and call 911 if appropriate, you then check the victim to see what problems may need first aid. This check, called an **assessment,** has three steps:

1. Check for responsiveness and immediate life-threatening conditions (check the ABCs).
2. Get the victim's history (find out what happened and what may have contributed to the emergency).
3. Check the rest of the victim's body (perform a physical examination).

While giving first aid and waiting for help to arrive, continue with a fourth step:

4. Monitor the victim for any changes.

Always perform these steps in this order. If there is an immediate life-threatening problem, such as stopped breathing, the victim needs immediate help. This victim could die if you first spent time looking for broken bones or asking bystanders what happened. ***Always remember:*** Check the ABCs first.

Check the ABCs

In less than a minute you can check the victim for immediate life-threatening conditions. This is called checking the ABCs where:

A = Airway

B = Breathing

C = Circulation

We need these three things functioning to stay alive.

Begin your check of the ABCs by speaking to the victim as you approach. **If the victim can speak or cough, then the airway is open, the victim is breathing, and the heart is beating.**

Unless the victim is obviously alert, **check for responsiveness.** Tap the victim on the shoulder and ask if he or she is okay. A victim is responsive if he or she speaks to you, moves purposefully, or otherwise responds to stimuli. A victim who does not respond is called unresponsive. An unresponsive victim is considered to have a potentially life-threatening condition. If the victim is unresponsive, continue checking the ABCs.

A = Airway

We can breathe only if our airway is open. The airway may be blocked by something stuck in the throat or by an unresponsive victim's own tongue. To make sure the tongue is not obstructing the airway in an unresponsive victim, position the victim's head to open the airway. In a victim not suspected of having a neck injury, tilt the head back and lift the chin as shown in Figure 2-1. This is called the head tilt-chin lift.

If the victim may have a neck or spine injury, do not tilt the head back to open the airway. Instead, only lift the jaw upward using both hands (**Figure 2-2**). This is called a jaw thrust. To perform the jaw thrust, position your thumbs on the apples of the victim's cheeks and your index and middle fingers on the jaw just below the ears. Provide gentle pressure with your index and middle fingers to move the jaw forward and the tongue away from the back of the throat.

B = Breathing

After opening the airway you then check to see if the victim is breathing. Lean over with your ear close to the person's mouth and nose and **look** at the victim's chest to see if it rises and falls with breathing. **Listen** for any sounds of breathing and **feel** for breath on your cheek. If you do not notice any signs of breathing within ten seconds, assume the person is not breathing.

At this point, using a barrier device if available (see Chapter 1), give two slow breaths to a victim who is not breathing. Watch for a rise and fall in the victim's chest to ensure your breath is entering the victim's lungs. If the breaths do not go in, attempt to reposition the airway to ensure it is open and try again. If the breaths still do not go in give care for choking (see Chapter 4).

C = Circulation

If the victim's airway is open and he or she is breathing, or you are breathing for the victim, you next check for circulation. This means checking that the heart is beating and blood is moving around the body (circulating). If the victim's heart has stopped or the victim is bleeding profusely, there is a circulation problem and the victim can die. **If the victim is moving, coughing, speaking, or breathing, the heart is beating.**

Check for signs of circulation by scanning the body for any signs of breathing, coughing, movement, and normal skin condition. Lack of circulation may be indicated by bluish, pale skin color, cool skin temperature, and clammy skin. It is currently recommended that *only healthcare workers or professional rescuers spend time checking for a victim's pulse.* Check for severe bleeding by quickly looking over the victim's body for obvious blood. Control any severe bleeding with direct pressure.

If you see no signs of circulation, start CPR and call for an automated external defibrillator (AED) to be brought to the scene (see Chapter 5).

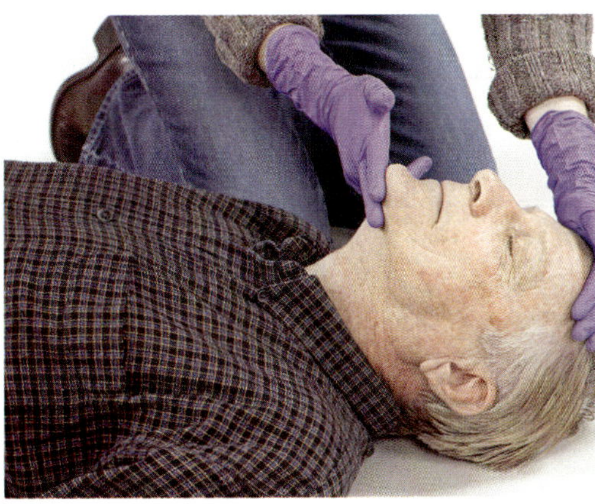

Figure 2-1 Head tilt-chin lift.

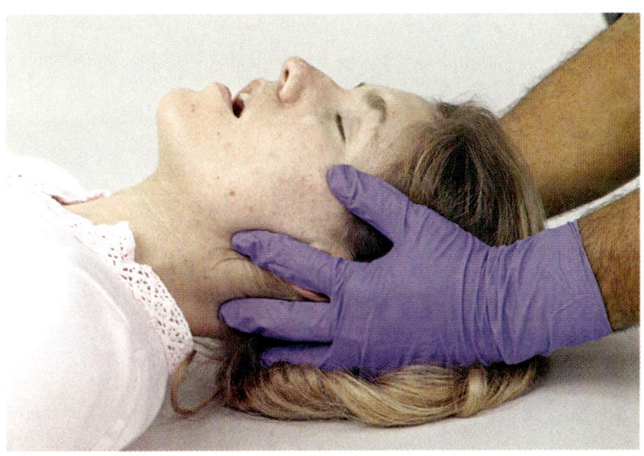

Figure 2-2 Jaw thrust.

Perform the Skill

Check the ABCs

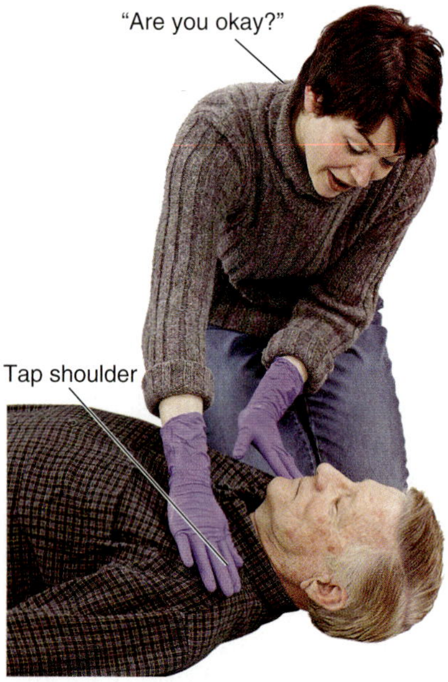

1 Check responsiveness.

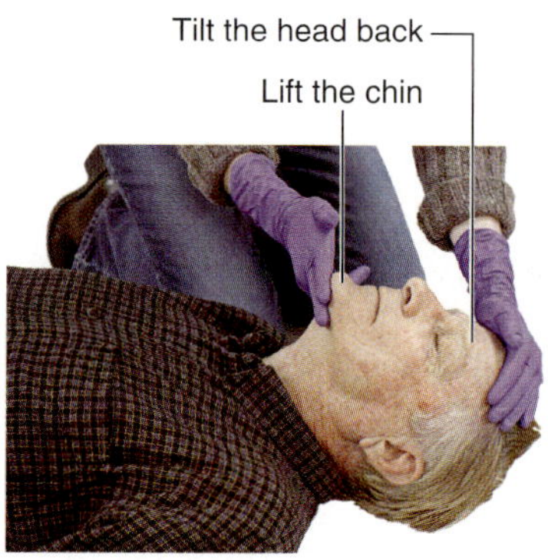

2 Open the airway.

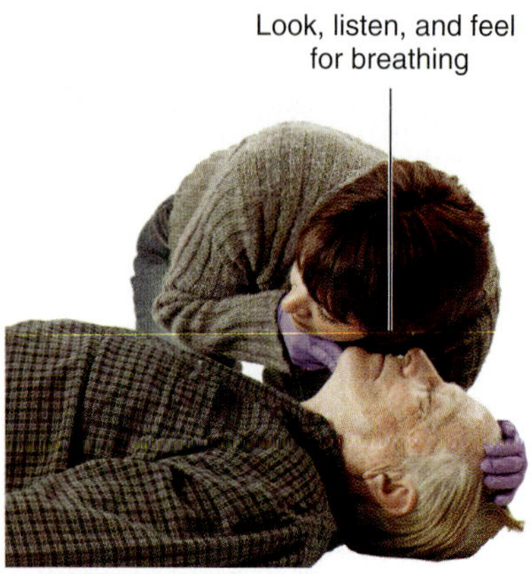

3 Check for breathing.

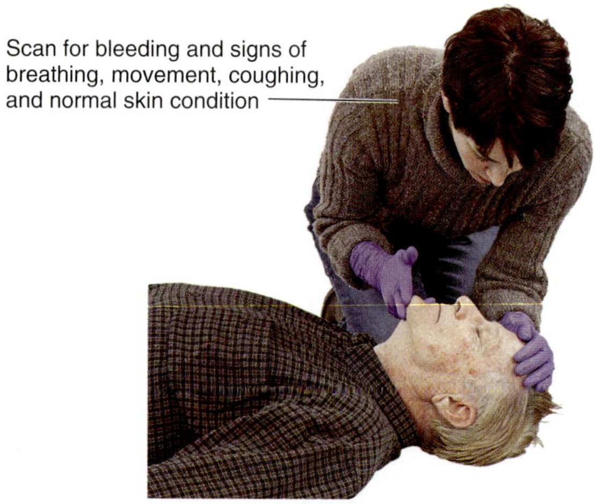

4 Check for signs of circulation.

Get the Victim's History

After checking the ABCs for immediate life-threatening conditions, try to find out more about what happened and the victim's condition. Talk to a responsive victim, or ask bystanders about what they know or saw in a situation involving an unresponsive victim. Use the **SAMPLE** history format:

S = ***Signs and symptoms.*** What can you observe about the victim (signs)? Ask the victim how he or she feels (symptoms).

A = ***Allergies.*** Ask the victim about any allergies to foods, medicines, insect stings, or other substances. Look for a medical alert bracelet.

M = ***Medications.*** Ask if the victim is taking any prescribed medications or over-the-counter products.

P = ***Previous problems.*** Ask the victim if he or she has had anything like this before or has any other illnesses.

L = ***Last food or drink.*** Ask the victim what and when he or she last ate or drank anything.

E = ***Events.*** Ask the victim what happened and try to identify the events that led to the current situation.

The information from a SAMPLE history may help you care for the victim. If the victim is unresponsive when help arrives, give any information gathered to the EMS professionals. It will help them to give the appropriate medical care.

Physical Examination

The third step of the assessment of an injured or ill victim is the physical examination. With this examination you may find other injuries that need first aid or additional clues to a victim's condition. Do not, however, stop giving first aid for a serious condition just to do or complete this examination. Instead, keep the victim still and calm and wait for EMS professionals to examine the victim.

This manual focuses on first aid given when there is a life-threatening problem with the victim's airway, breathing or circulation. First aiders who want more information on other injuries and the complete physical assessment are encouraged to take the National Safety Council course on Basic First Aid (www.nsc.org).

Monitor the Victim

In cases of serious or life-threatening illness or injury, you should have called 911. While waiting for help to arrive, monitor the victim to make sure his or her condition does not worsen. With an unresponsive victim or a victim with a serious injury, repeat your assessment of the ABCs at least every five minutes. Stay prepared to give CPR or other care if needed.

Learning Checkpoint 1

1. You first encounter a victim lying quietly on the floor. Number the following actions in the correct order.

_____ **a.** Check victim for signs of circulation

_____ **b.** Listen near victim's mouth for breathing sounds

_____ **c.** Check to see if victim responds to your voice or touch

_____ **d.** Open the victim's airway

2. Describe three ways you can detect if a victim is breathing.

____

3. True or False: If you hear a victim coughing or breathing, you can assume the heart is beating.

4. Write what each letter in the SAMPLE history stands for:

S = _______________

A = _______________

M = _______________

P = _______________

L = _______________

E = _______________

Chapter

3 Cardiac Emergencies

CHAPTER PREVIEW

- Heart Attack
- Angina

Many different illnesses may occur suddenly and become medical emergencies. Recognizing the signs and symptoms of such things as heart attack and angina may help you give life-saving care sooner.

Heart Attack

Heart attack is a sudden reduced blood flow to the heart muscle. It is a medical emergency because it can lead to **cardiac arrest** (a sudden stop in the beating of the heart). Heart attack can occur at any age. The signs and symptoms of heart attack vary considerably, from vague chest discomfort (which the victim may confuse with heartburn) to crushing pain, with or without other symptoms. The victim may have no signs and symptoms at all before collapsing suddenly. Often the victim has milder symptoms that come and go for two or three days before the heart attack occurs. It is important to consider the possibility of heart attack with a wide range of symptoms rather than expecting a clearly defined situation (**Figure 3-1**).

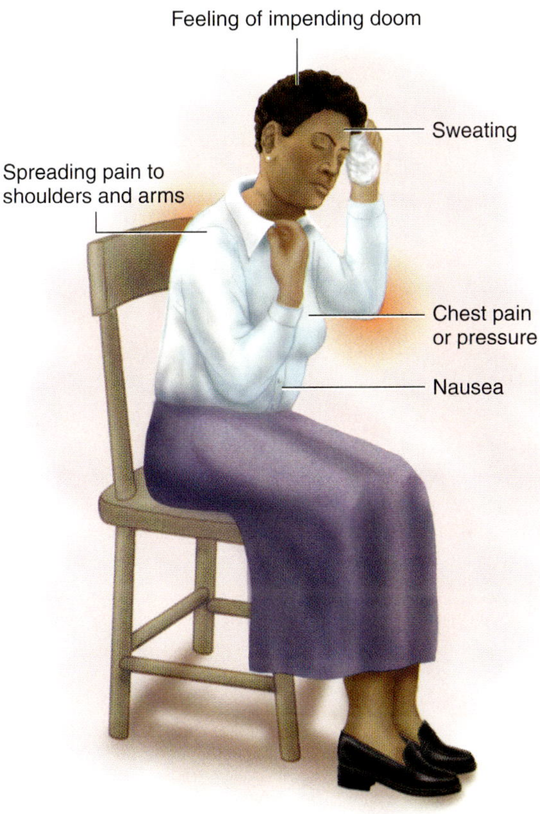

Figure 3-1 Signs and symptoms of a heart attack.

FACTS ABOUT HEART ATTACK

- Half a million people a year in the U.S. die from heart attacks—many of whom could have been saved by prompt CPR, AED use, and medical treatment.
- Heart attack results from coronary artery disease, which can often be prevented or minimized with a healthy diet, exercise, not smoking, and regular medical care.
- Heart attack is more likely in those with a family history of heart attacks.
- One-fifth of heart attack victims do not have chest pain—but often have other symptoms.
- Heart attack victims typically deny that they are having a heart attack. Don't let the victim talk you out of getting help!

When You See

- Complaints of persistent pressure, tightness, ache, or pain in the chest
- Pain may spread to neck, shoulders, or arms
- Shortness of breath
- Dizziness, lightheadedness, feeling of impending doom
- Pale skin, sweating
- Nausea

Do This First

1. Call 911 immediately, even if the victim says it is not serious.
2. Help the victim rest in a comfortable position. Loosen constricting clothing.
3. Allow the victim to take one aspirin (unless allergic).
4. Stay with the victim, be reassuring and calming, and be prepared to give CPR if needed (see Chapter 4).

Additional Care

- Ask the victim if he or she is taking heart medication, and help obtain the medication
- Do not let the victim eat or drink anything

Angina

Angina is a chest pain caused by heart disease that usually happens after intense activity or exertion. The pain usually lasts only a few minutes. People usually know when they have angina and may carry medication for it.

Help a person with angina take his or her own medication and rest. If the pain persists more than ten minutes or stops and then returns, or if the victim has other heart attack symptoms, give first aid as for a heart attack.

Learning Checkpoint 1

1. True or False: Heart attacks occur only in people over age 50.
2. What are the signs and symptoms of heart attack? (Check all that apply.)
   - _____ Persistent pressure or pain in the chest
   - _____ Bright red rash on chest over heart
   - _____ Shortness of breath
   - _____ Dizziness, lightheadedness
   - _____ Frequent need to urinate
   - _____ Pale skin, sweating
   - _____ Nausea
3. Steps to take for a victim having a heart attack include: (Check all that apply.)
   - _____ Call 911 immediately
   - _____ Give the victim lots of fluids to drink
   - _____ Help the victim rest in a comfortable position
   - _____ Allow the victim to take one aspirin (unless allergic)
   - _____ Massage victim's legs vigorously
   - _____ Be prepared to give CPR if needed
4. True or False: A person who takes medication for angina can never have a heart attack.

Chapter

4 Basic Life Support

CHAPTER PREVIEW

- Recovery Position
- Rescue Breathing
- Choking
- CPR

Basic life support (BLS) refers to first aid given if the victim's breathing or heart stops. Many things can cause breathing or the heart to stop. BLS is often needed for victims of

- Heart attack
- Drowning
- Choking
- Other injuries or conditions that affect breathing or the heart

OVERVIEW OF BLS

Giving BLS involves one or more life-saving skills, depending on the victim's needs. These skills are sometimes called **resuscitation** and include:

- ***Rescue breathing*** to get needed oxygen into the lungs
- ***Chest compressions*** to pump oxygenated blood to vital organs
- Use of an ***automated external defibrillator (AED)*** to shock the heart to beat regularly
- ***Choking care,*** including chest compressions, to expel an obstructing object from the airway

Differences Among Adults, Children, and Infants

Because of size and other differences, there are some distinctions in how BLS skills are used with adults, children, and infants. These differences are described later in this chapter and are based on age. Standard age groups are defined in the following way:

Infant — birth to 1 year
Child — ages 1 to 8
Adult — over age 8

Cardiac Chain of Survival

Although BLS includes care given to any victim whose breathing or circulation stops, cardiac arrest victims are a common type of victim needing BLS. Causes of sudden cardiac arrest include such things as:

- Heart attack
- Certain heart medications
- Drug abuse or overdose
- Electrocution, drowning, choking, traumatic injury

To recognize the urgent need for quick actions to save the lives of cardiac arrest victims, the Citizen CPR Foundation created the concept of the cardiac **chain of survival** (**Figure 4-1**). This chain has four crucial links:

1. ***Early Access.*** Recognize that a victim whose heart has stopped *needs help immediately!*

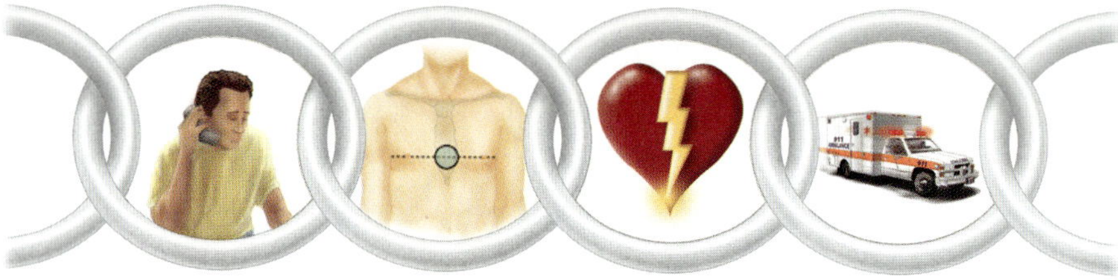

Figure 4-1 Cardiac chain of survival.

However, you must also be able to recognize the signs and symptoms of a potential life-threatening injury such as a heart attack in a responsive person (see Chapter 3). Do not wait until a person becomes unresponsive to start the chain of events needed to keep the victim alive. Call 911 and get help on the way.

2. ***Early CPR.*** For a victim without signs of circulation (breathing, coughing, movement, normal skin condition), start cardiopulmonary resuscitation (CPR) immediately. This helps keep the brain and other vital organs supplied with oxygen until help arrives.
3. ***Early Defibrillation.*** An AED, now present in many public and work places, can help get the heart beating normally again after a cardiac arrest. Send someone right away to get the AED.
4. ***Early Advanced Care.*** The sooner the victim is treated by emergency care professionals, the better the chance for survival. You can help make sure the victim reaches this last link in the chain by acting immediately with the earlier links.

The Recovery Position

An unresponsive victim who is breathing when found or after receiving BLS should be put in the recovery position (**Figure 4-2**). This position:

- Helps keep the airway open
- Allows fluids to drain from the mouth
- Prevents inhaling stomach contents if the victim vomits

Once in the recovery position, continue to monitor the victim's breathing.

Rescue Breathing

Rescue breathing is used with any nonbreathing victim to get needed oxygen into the person's lungs. Start rescue breathing immediately when you check the ABCs and discover the victim is not breathing. See "Perform the Skill: Rescue Breathing for Adults and Children" for the steps to take.

Since a victim who is not breathing may be in cardiac arrest, have someone call 911 immediately, and if an AED is available, send someone to get it.

ALERT

Rescue Breathing

Do not blow harder than is needed to make the victim's chest rise.
After the breath remember to let the air escape and the chest fall.
Blowing in too forcefully or for too long is ineffective and may put air in the stomach, which may cause vomiting.

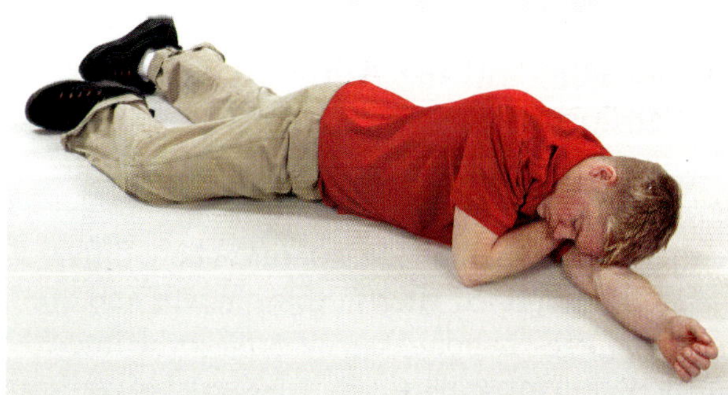

Figure 4-2 The recovery position.

Perform the Skill

Recovery Position

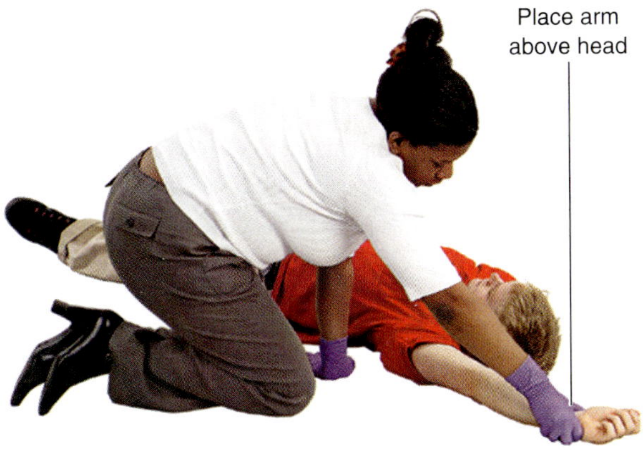

1 Position the victim's arm.

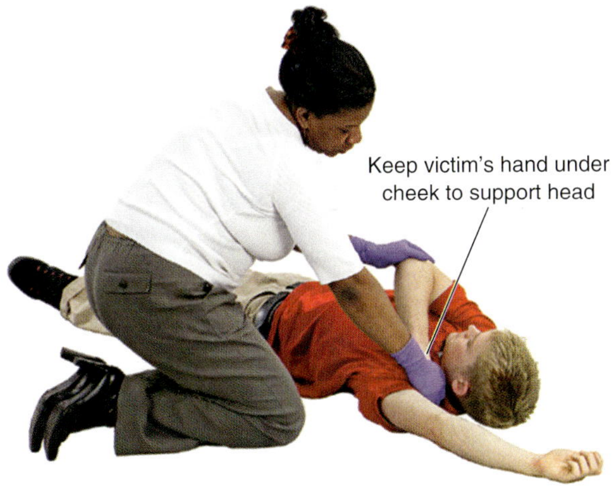

2 Move victim's other arm across chest and against cheek.

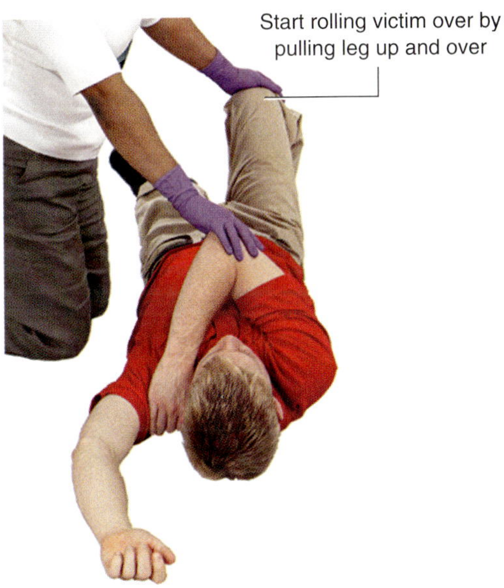

3 Bend the victim's leg at the knee and pull it toward you as you roll the victim onto his or her side.

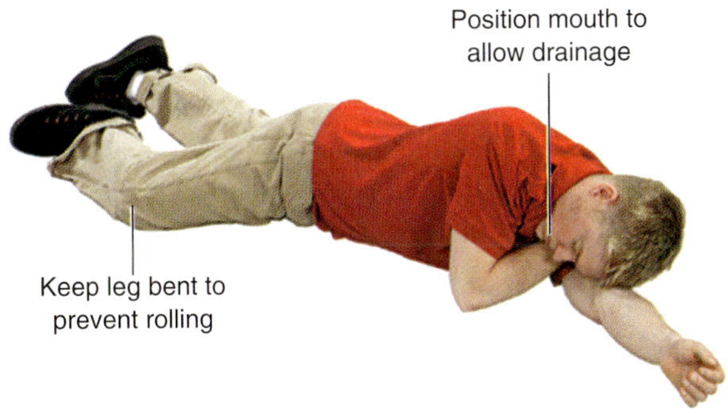

4 Adjust victim's position as needed.

Techniques of Rescue Breathing

To begin rescue breathing position the victim on his or her back and open the airway using either the head tilt-chin lift or the jaw thrust (see Chapter 2). Use a barrier device if you have one but do not delay rescue breathing to get one. With all techniques of rescue breathing, watch the victim's chest rise to make sure your air is going into the lungs.

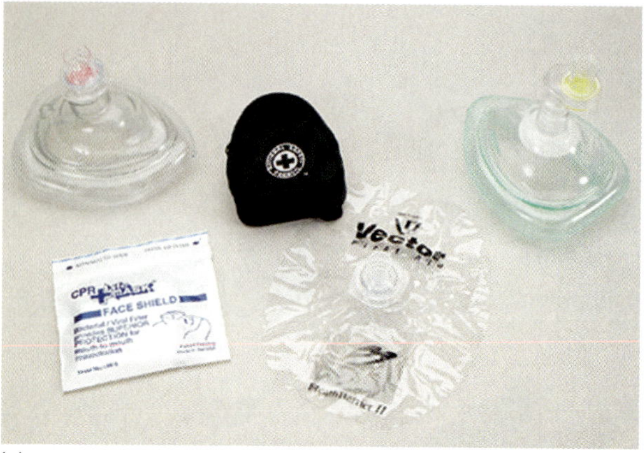

(a)

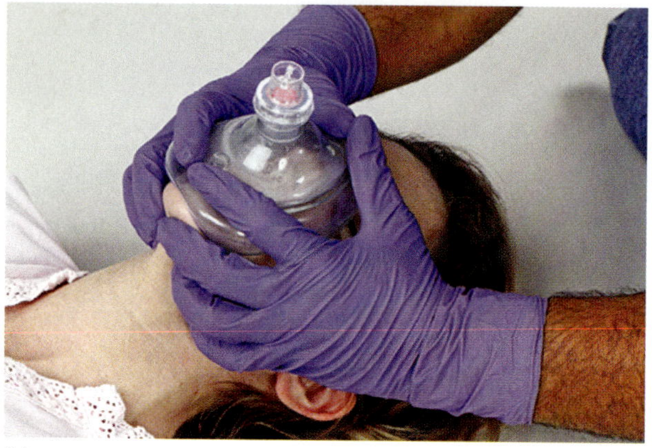

(b)

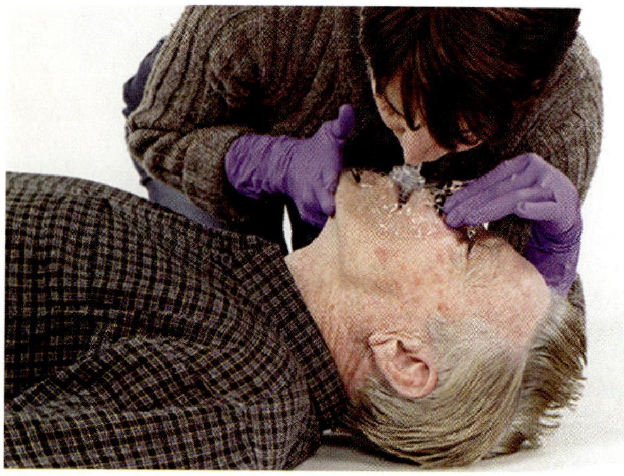

(c)

Figure 4-3 (a) Barrier devices. (b) Position pocket mask over mouth and nose. (c) Position barrier device over mouth and pinch nose.

Mouth to Barrier

Barrier devices are always recommended when giving rescue breathing. Position a pocket mask or face shield on the victim's face and give breaths through the device. Make sure it is sealed to the victim's face and your air is going into the victim. When using a face shield, pinch the victim's nose closed when giving a breath (**Figure 4-3**).

Mouth to Mouth

If you do not have a barrier device, pinch the victim's nose shut and seal your mouth over the victim's mouth. Breathe into the victim's mouth, watching the chest rise to confirm the air going in.

Mouth to Nose

Give rescue breathing through the victim's nose if the mouth cannot be opened or is injured, or if you cannot get a good seal with your mouth over the victim's. Hold the victim's mouth closed, seal your mouth over the nose to breathe in, then let the mouth open to let the air escape.

Mouth to Stoma

Because of past illness or injury, some people breathe through a hole in their lower neck called a stoma. During your check of the ABCs check this hole to see if the victim is breathing. Cup your hand over the victim's nose and mouth, seal your barrier device (or your mouth) over the stoma, and give rescue breaths as usual (**Figure 4-4**).

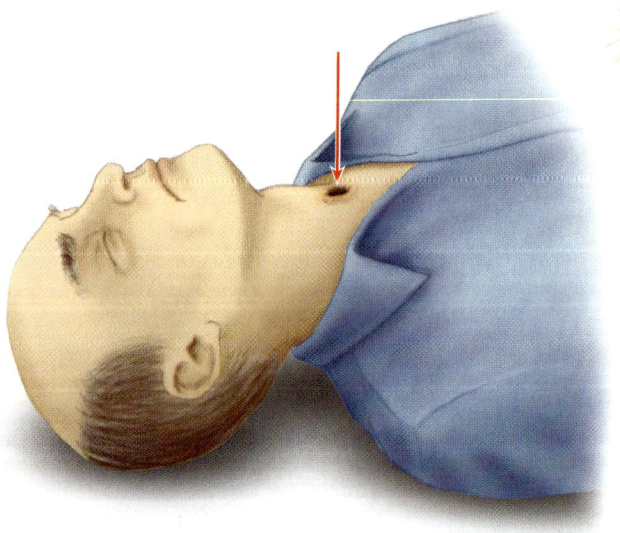

Figure 4-4 Victim with a stoma.

Perform the Skill

Rescue Breathing for Adults and Children

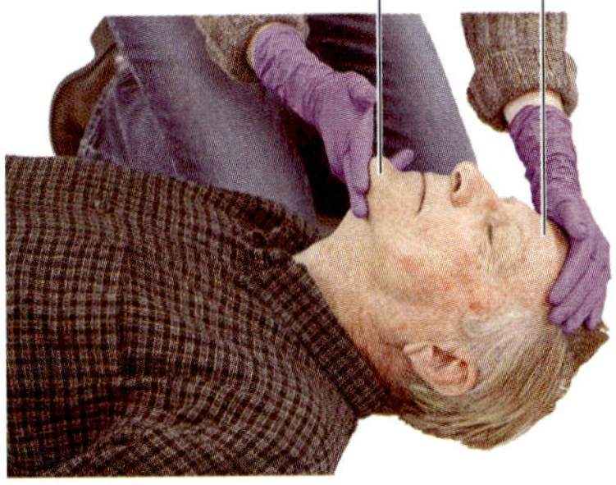

1 Open the airway. Look, listen, and feel for breathing for up to 10 seconds.

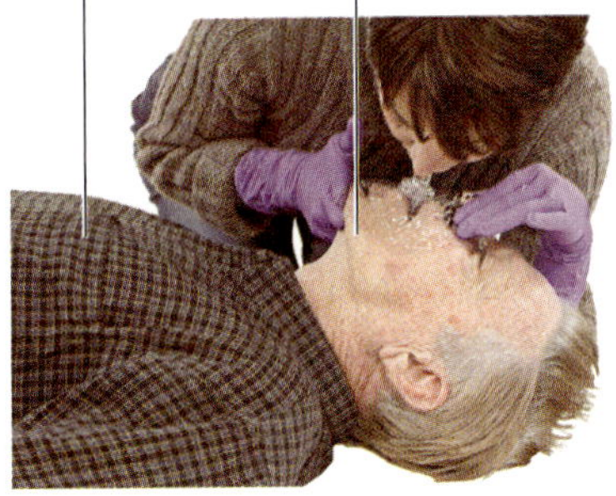

2 If not breathing, give 2 slow breaths (2 seconds each for adults, 1–1½ seconds each for children), watching chest rise and letting it fall.

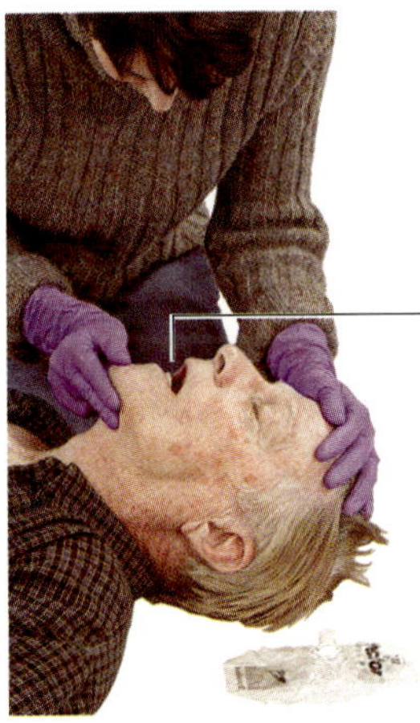

3 If your breaths do not go in, try again to open the airway and give two more rescue breaths. If they still do not go in, the victim may be choking. Proceed to CPR.

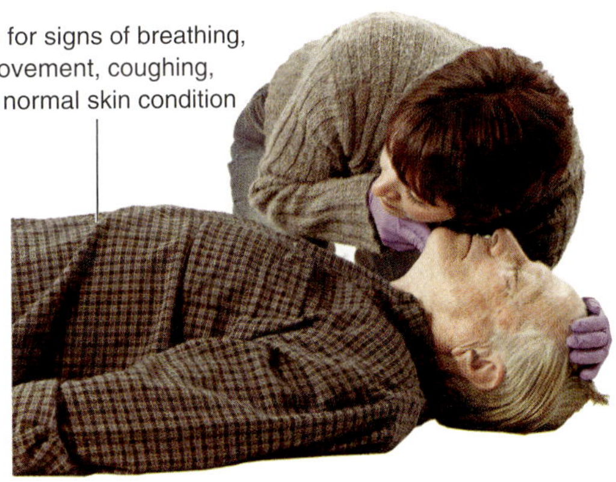

4 If your first 2 breaths go in, check victim for signs of circulation. If there are signs of circulation but no breathing, continue rescue breathing at rate of 1 breath every 5 seconds for adult (1 breath every 3 seconds for child). If there are no signs of circulation, start CPR.

Infants

Rescue breathing for infants is similar to that for adults and children, with these differences:

- Gently tilt the head back to open the airway and check breathing—do not overextend the neck
- Cover both the mouth and nose with your mouth to give breaths. (Use the mouth or nose only if you cannot cover both.)
- Give breaths lasting 1–1½ seconds each (instead of 2 with adults)

Learning Checkpoint 1

1. Basic life support helps keep a victim alive if the __________ or _________ has stopped.

2. Rescue breathing is needed to:

a. Get oxygen into the victim's blood

b. Circulate the blood to vital organs

c. Open the victim's airway

d. All of the above

3. For purposes of basic life support techniques, a child is defined as someone between the ages of ____ and _____.

4. Number in correct order the links in the cardiac chain of survival:

_____ Early defibrillation

_____ Early access

_____ Early CPR

_____ Early advanced care

5. Describe the steps for putting an adult or child in the recovery position.

____

6. True or False: Blow as hard as you can into the victim's mouth during rescue breathing.

7. What is the best way to confirm your breaths are going into the victim's lungs?

a. Listen at the victim's mouth for escaping air

b. Place one hand on the victim's abdomen to feel movement

c. Watch the victim's chest rise and fall

d. None of the above

Choking (Airway Obstruction)

Choking is a total or partial obstruction of the airway by a foreign object. It occurs commonly in infants and small children who put objects in their mouths, and in children or adults when eating. With a total obstruction, the victim becomes unresponsive within minutes. CPR is given to an unresponsive victim because the chest thrusts may expel the foreign object (see Cardiopulmonary Resuscitation (CPR) section later in this chapter).

Perform the Skill

Care for Choking Adults and Children

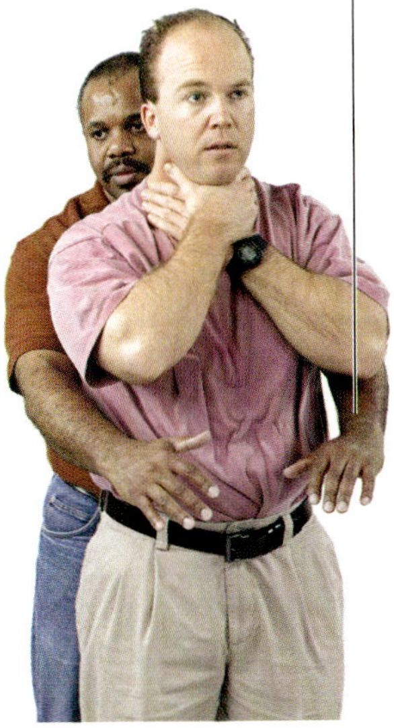

1 Stand behind the victim and reach around the abdomen.

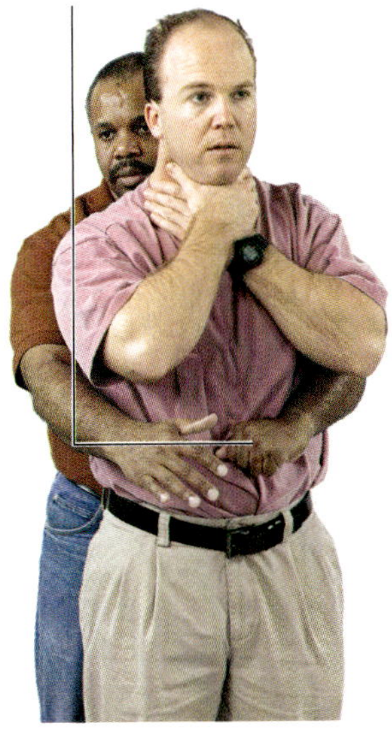

2 Make a fist with one hand and grasp it with the other (thumb side into abdomen).

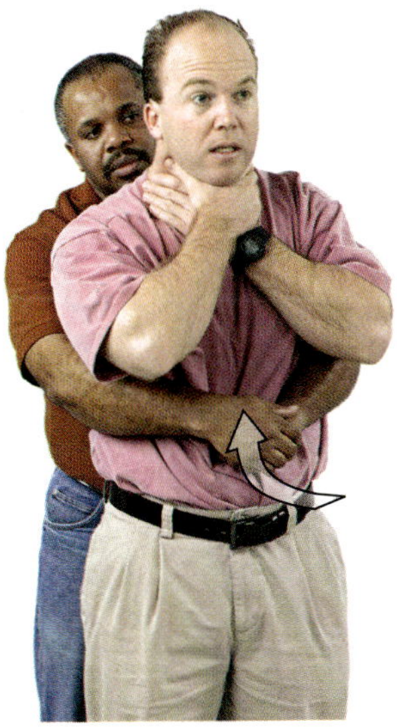

3 Thrust inward and upward into the abdomen with quick jerks. Continue until the victim can expel the object or becomes unresponsive.

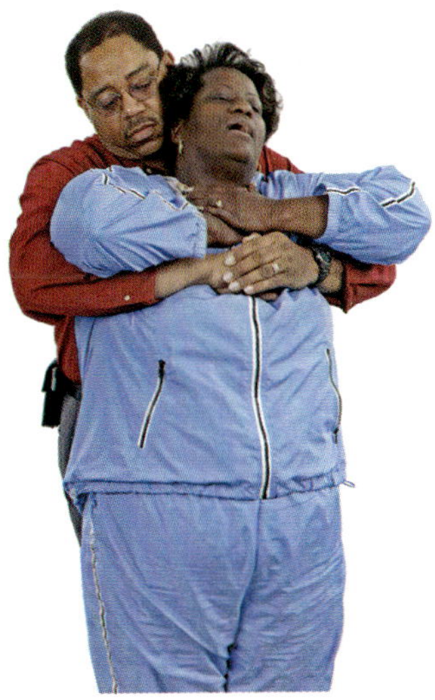

4 For a responsive pregnant victim, or any victim you cannot get your arms around, give chest thrusts.

Care for Choking Adults and Children

When You See

In a responsive adult or child victim:

- Coughing, wheezing, difficulty breathing
- Clutching at throat
- Pale or bluish coloring around mouth and nailbeds

Do This First

1. If victim is coughing, encourage continued coughing to clear the object.
2. If not coughing, ask if victim can breathe or speak. If not, get victim's consent and give abdominal thrusts (Heimlich maneuver).
3. If the victim becomes unresponsive, start CPR. If you are alone, call 911 after 1 minute.

Additional Care

- For a responsive pregnant victim or any victim you cannot get your arms around, give chest thrusts instead of abdominal thrusts

Perform the Skill

Choking in an Infant

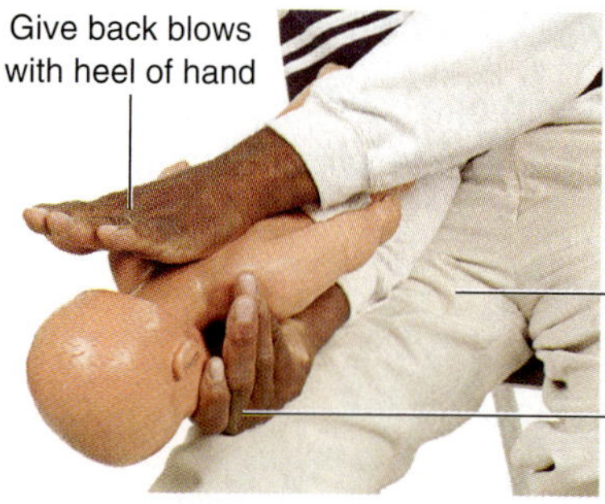

1 Support the infant's head in one hand, with the torso on your forearm and your thigh. Give up to 5 back blows between the shoulder blades.

2 Check for object expelled. If not present, continue with next step.

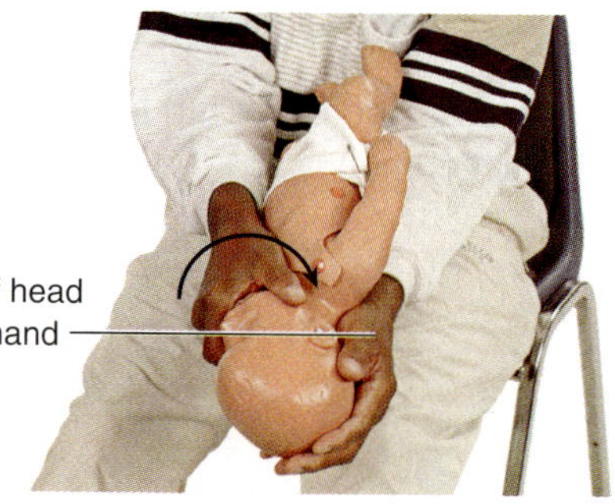

3 With other hand on back of infant's head, roll the infant face up.

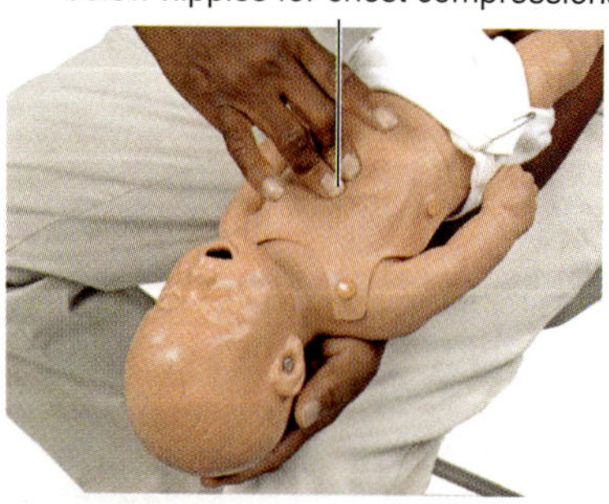

4 Give up to 5 chest thrusts with middle and ring fingers. Check mouth for expelled object.

5 Repeat steps 1-4, alternating back blows and chest thrusts and checking the mouth. If alone, call 911 after 1 minute. Continue until object is expelled or the infant becomes unresponsive.

6 If the infant becomes unresponsive, give CPR.

Self-Treating Choking

If you are choking when alone, give yourself abdominal thrusts to try to expel the object. You may try using your hands, or lean over and push your abdomen against the back of a chair or other firm object (**Figure 4-5**).

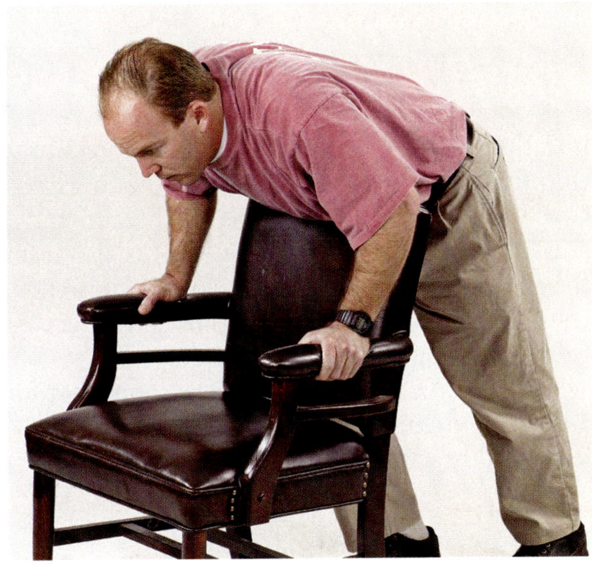

Figure 4-5 Abdominal self-thrusts.

Care for Choking Infants

If a choking infant can cry or cough, watch carefully to see if the object comes out. If the infant cannot cry or cough, follow the steps for back blows and chest thrusts in "Perform the Skill: Choking in an Infant." If the infant becomes unresponsive, send someone to call 911, and give CPR. Check for an object in the mouth before you give a breath, and sweep out any object you see with one finger.

Learning Checkpoint 2

1. For a responsive adult victim who is choking:

a. Start CPR immediately

b. Slap the victim hard on the back

c. Give abdominal thrusts

d. No first aid action is needed until the victim becomes unresponsive

2. True or False: A choking victim who is coughing is still able to breathe and may be able to cough out the foreign object.

3. True or False: A choking victim who is unable to breathe will soon become unresponsive and the heart will stop.

4. For a responsive choking infant:

a. Support the head as you position the infant

b. Alternate back blows and chest thrusts

c. Check the infant's mouth for an expelled object

d. All of the above

5. Explain why CPR is given to a choking victim who becomes unresponsive.

____

Cardiopulmonary Resuscitation (CPR)

CPR combines rescue breathing (to get oxygen into the victim's lungs) with chest compressions (to pump the oxygenated blood to vital organs). Give CPR to any victim who is not breathing and has no signs of circulation. CPR is also used for an unresponsive choking victim because the chest compressions can expel a foreign object from the victim's airway.

The specific steps for CPR vary somewhat for adults, children, and infants. It is important to learn and practice the skills for all age groups.

Call First/Call Fast

If someone else is present at the scene, have that person call 911 as soon as you recognize a victim is unresponsive. Shout for any bystanders who may hear you, and have them call 911 and go for an AED. If you are alone, follow these guidelines to *call first* versus *call fast*. In some circumstances it is important to start the process of getting an AED to the victim first before starting CPR.

Call first for:

- Unresponsive adult victim
- Infant or child with known heart problem seen to collapse suddenly

Call fast (after giving 1 minute of care) for:

- Unresponsive child or infant (0–8 years)
- Adult victim of near-drowning, poisoning, drug overdose, or traumatic injury

Technique of CPR

CPR alternates giving chest compressions and rescue breaths. After checking the victim's ABCs and determining there are no signs of breathing or circulation, start chest compressions after giving the initial two breaths. For a victim of any age, these are the general steps of CPR:

1. Find the correct hand position on the lower half of the breastbone midway between the nipples (**Figure 4-6**).
2. Compress the chest quickly and rhythmically at a rate of at least 100 compressions per minute for an infant, or 100 compressions per minute for an adult or child.
3. Alternate chest compressions and rescue breaths in the correct ratio for adult or infant/child.

For the detailed CPR steps, see "Perform the Skill: CPR for Adults and Children" and "Perform the Skill: CPR for Infants." Here are the primary CPR differences depending on the victim's age:

CPR Essentials

Adults	Children	Infants
Compression:		
heels of both hands	heel of one hand	two middle fingers
Chest depth:		
1½ to 2 inches	1 to 1½ inches	½ to 1 inch
Compressions to breaths:		
15 to 2	5 to 1	5 to 1

Note that the chest compression depth is roughly 1/3 of the depth of the victim's body. This may help you ensure your chest compressions are deep enough to be effective.

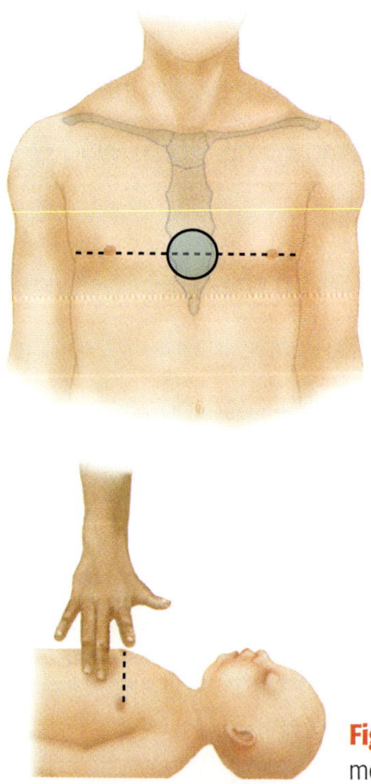

Figure 4-6 Proper placement for compressions.

Perform the Skill

CPR for Adults and Children

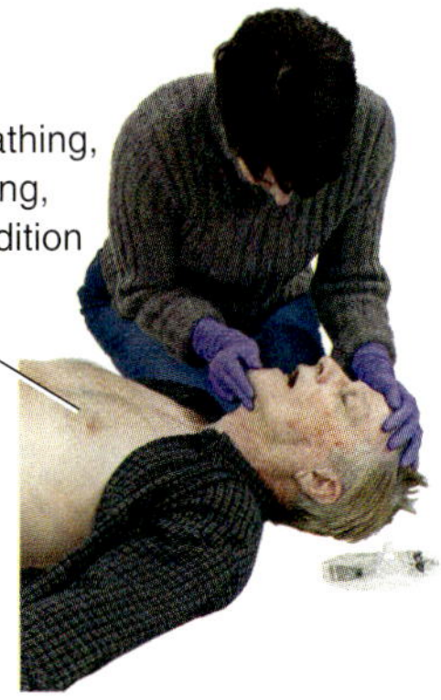

1 Open airway and determine the victim is not breathing.

2 Give 2 rescue breaths (2 seconds each for adult; 1–1$^1/_2$ seconds each for child).

3 Determine victim has no signs of circulation.

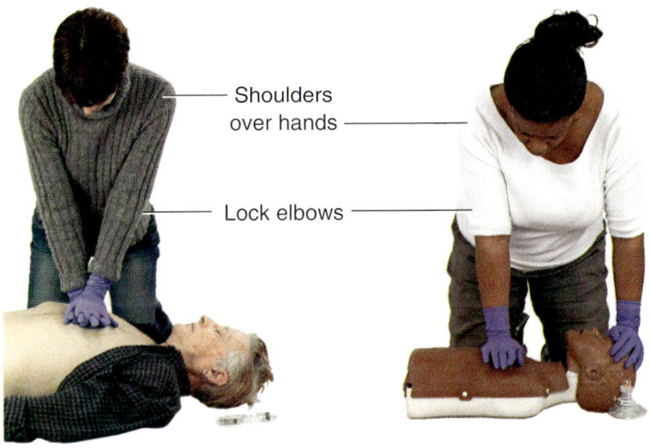

4 Put hand in correct position for chest compressions. For adult, put second hand on top of first and interlock fingers.

5 Give 15 chest compressions 1$^1/_2$–2 inches deep in an adult (5 compressions 1–1$^1/_2$ inches deep in a child) at rate of 100 per minute. Count aloud for a steady fast rate: "One, two, three. . . ." Then give 2 breaths (one breath for a child).

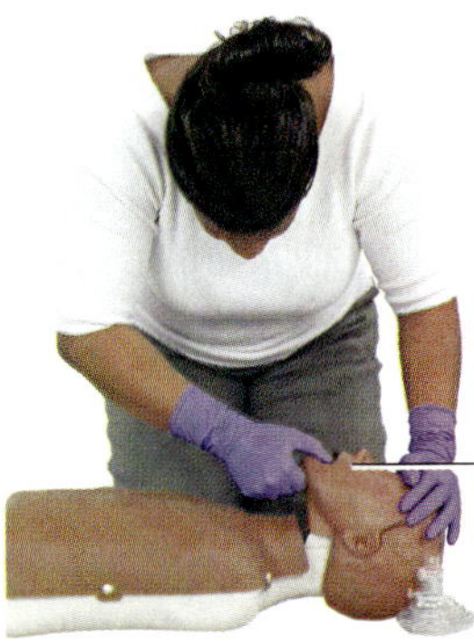

6 Continue cycles of 15 compressions and 2 breaths in adult (5 compressions and 1 breath in child). If the victim may have been choking, look inside mouth when opening the mouth to give breaths, and remove any object by sweeping it out with your finger.

7 After 1 minute of CPR, pause and check the victim again for signs of circulation. If absent, continue with chest compressions and rescue breaths. Then check again every few minutes.

(continued)

Perform the Skill

CPR for Adults and Children

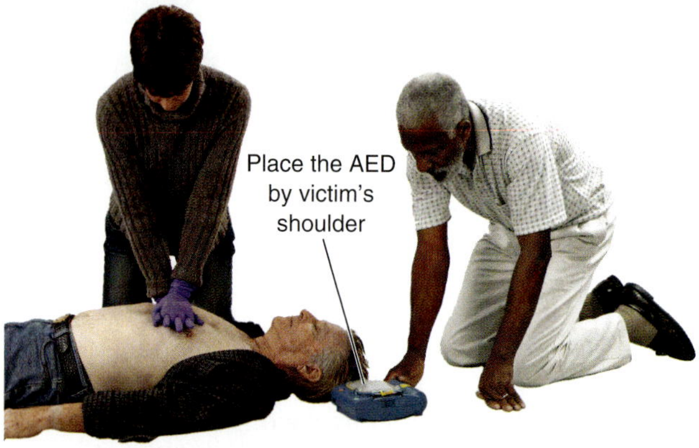

8 Continue CPR until:
- Victim shows signs of circulation or breathing
- An AED is brought to the scene and is ready to use
- Help arrives and takes over
- You are too exhausted to continue

9 a. If the victim starts breathing and has signs of circulation, put in the recovery position and monitor his or her condition.

b. If the victim has signs of circulation but is not breathing, continue giving rescue breaths at a rate of 1 every 5 seconds (every 3 seconds for a child).

c. If the victim has no signs of circulation, continue with CPR. When an AED arrives, start the AED sequence.

ALERT

Chest Compressions

Be careful with your hand position for chest compressions. Do not give compressions over the bottom tip of the breastbone. When compressing, keep your elbows straight and keep your hands in contact with the chest at all times.

Compression-Only CPR

A nonbreathing victim with no signs of circulation needs both rescue breathing and chest compressions to move oxygenated blood to vital organs. However, if for any reason you cannot or will not give rescue breathing, still give the victim chest compressions. This gives the victim a better chance for survival than doing nothing.

Perform the Skill

CPR for Infants

1 Open the airway and determine the infant is not breathing.

2 Give 2 rescue breaths (1–1½ seconds each).

3 Determine the infant has no signs of circulation.

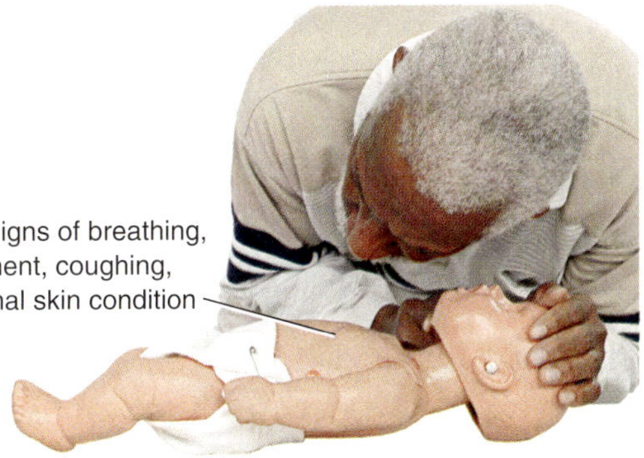

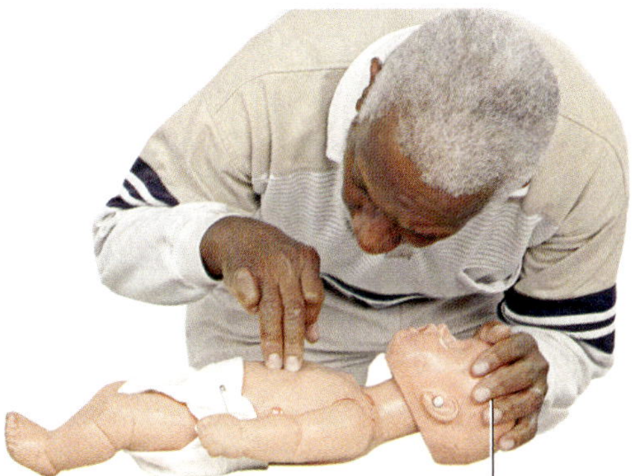

4 Put your 2 middle fingers about one finger-width below an imaginary line between the nipples for chest compressions.

5 Give 5 chest compressions ½–1 inch deep at rate of at least 100 per minute. Count aloud for a steady fast rate: "One, two, three…." Then give another breath.

6 Continue cycles of 5 compressions followed by 1 breath. If the infant may have been choking, look inside the mouth when opening it to give rescue breaths.

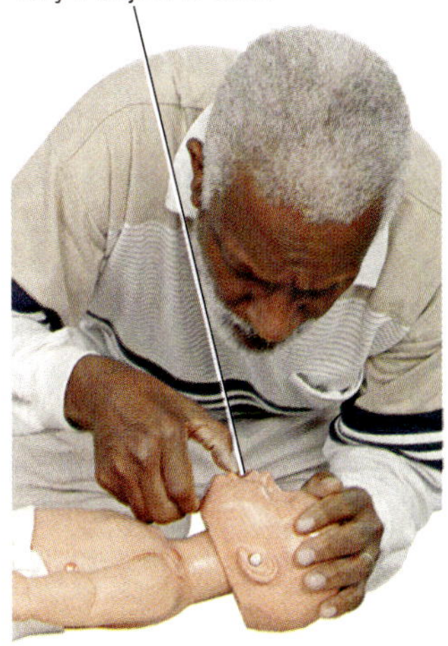

7 After 1 minute of CPR, pause and check the victim again for signs of circulation, then continue with chest compressions and rescue breaths. Check again every few minutes.

8 Continue CPR until:
- Infant shows signs of circulation or breathing
- Help arrives and takes over
- You are too exhausted to continue

9 a. If the infant starts breathing and has signs of circulation, hold the infant and monitor his or her condition.
b. If the victim has signs of circulation but is not breathing, continue giving rescue breaths at a rate of 1 every 3 seconds.

Learning Checkpoint 3

1. CPR stands for:

   a. Cardiac position for recovery
   b. Cardiopulmonary resuscitation
   c. Chest pump rescue
   d. None of the above

2. *Call first* (before starting CPR) for which of these victims? (Check all that apply)

   _____ Unresponsive adult victim collapsed from unknown cause
   _____ Unresponsive infant
   _____ Unresponsive child with known heart problem
   _____ Unresponsive adult victim of near-drowning

3. When is it appropriate to start CPR?

   a. As soon as you determine the victim is unresponsive
   b. As soon as you determine the victim is not breathing
   c. As soon as you determine the victim is not breathing and has no signs of circulation
   d. Only when you have called 911 and the dispatcher tells you to start CPR

4. Describe how to find the site for chest compressions in an adult or child victim.

   ____

5. Chest compressions in an adult should be ___ to ___ inches deep. In a child, compress to a depth of ___ to ___ inches. In an infant, to a depth of ___ to ___ inch.

6. What is the correct ratio of chest compressions to breaths in an adult?

   a. 5 to 1
   b. 5 to 2
   c. 15 to 1
   d. 15 to 2

7. If you are performing CPR on an adult victim when an AED is brought to the scene and is ready to use, what action should you take?

   a. Use the AED immediately
   b. Continue CPR for at least 15 cycles before using the AED
   c. Use the AED only if you can feel the victim's heart quivering in the chest
   d. Use the AED only if the victim showed signs and symptoms of having a heart attack; otherwise, do not use it but continue CPR

Chapter

5 Using an Automated External Defibrillator

CHAPTER PREVIEW

- How AEDs Work
- Using an AED
- Special AED Considerations
- Potential AED Problems
- AED Maintenance

Not every victim who receives basic life support (BLS) needs an automated external defibrillator (AED), but many do. Remember the chain of survival. An AED should be used with a victim who is not breathing and has no signs of circulation. In cases of cardiac arrest the AED may restart a normal heartbeat.

Public Access to Defibrillation

Public access to defibrillation (PAD) programs have worked to make AEDs available in workplaces, public gathering places, and other facilities for use by trained rescuers and first aiders. In most areas a healthcare provider oversees placement and use of the AED, and your AED training must meet certain requirements. For professional rescuers, this is called **medical direction.** Your course instructor will inform you how to meet the legal requirements in your area for using an AED.

How AEDs Work

The heart functions to pump blood to the lungs to pick up oxygen and then pump oxygenated blood to all parts of the body. The heart consists of four chambers called the left atrium, the right atrium, and the left and right ventricles. The ventricles, the lower chambers of the heart, do most of the pumping. The heart's electrical system keeps the four chambers of the heart synchronized and working together. The sinus and atrioventricular (AV) nodes help organize and control the rhythmic electrical impulses that keep the heart beating properly (**Figure 5-1**).

With a heart attack or other heart problems, this rhythmic electrical control may be disrupted, causing an abnormal heart rhythm.

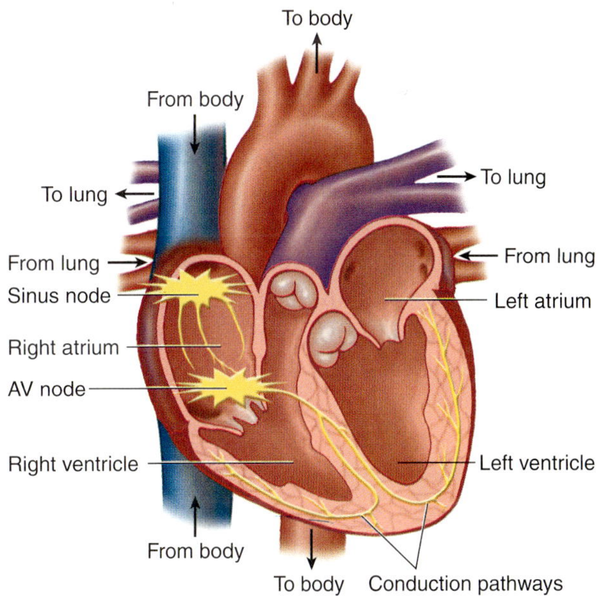

Figure 5-1 The heart.

Ventricular Fibrillation

Ventricular fibrillation (V-fib) is an abnormal heart rhythm that commonly occurs during heart attacks and stops circulation of the blood. Although we say a victim in V-fib is in **cardiac arrest,** the heart is not actually completely still, but is beating abnormally. **Fibrillation** means the ventricles of the heart are quivering instead of beating rhythmically. Blood is not filling the ventricles and is not being pumped out to the lungs or body as normal.

What the AED Does

The AED automatically checks the victim's heart rhythm and advises whether the victim needs a shock. If the victim's heart is in V-fib, the machine will advise giving an electric shock to return the heart to a normal rhythm. This is called **defibrillation,** or stopping the fibrillation of the heart (**Figure 5-2**).

Current AEDs are easy and simple to use, but they must be used right away. With every minute that goes by before defibrillation begins, the victim's chances for survival drop by about 10%.

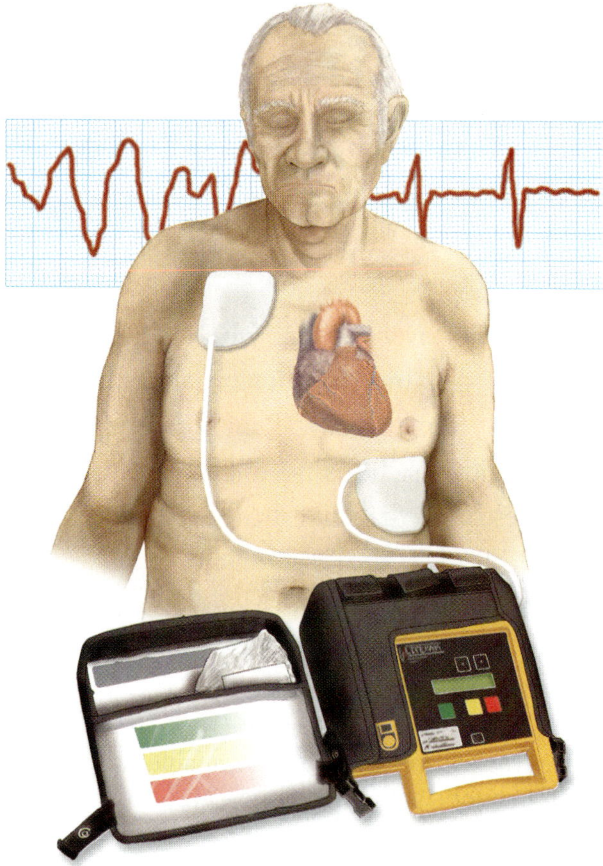

Figure 5-2 An AED gives a shock to the heart.

The AED

AEDs are complex inside but simple to use. They contain a battery and are portable. The unit has two pads connected to it with cables. These pads are placed on the victim's chest. The unit then analyzes the victim's heart and advises whether to give a shock. Some models have a screen that tells you what to do; all models give directions in a clear voice. AED models vary somewhat in other features, but all work in the same basic way (**Figure 5-3**).

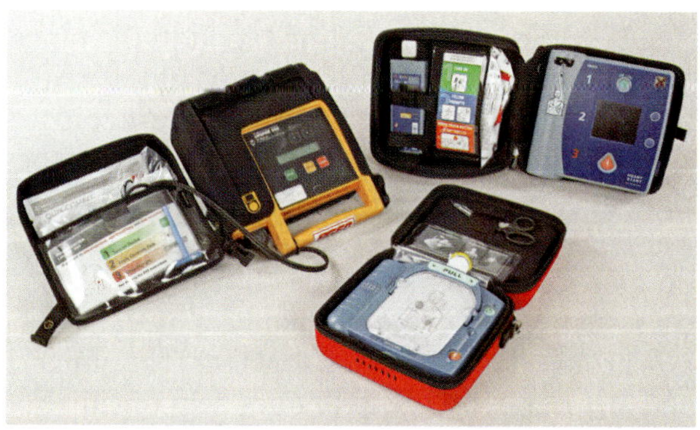

Figure 5-3 A variety of AEDs.

Using an AED

In any situation in which a victim suddenly collapses or is found unresponsive, be thinking about the possibility of cardiac arrest even as you come up to the victim. If someone else is present and you know an AED is available, send that person to get it *now*. It is better to have it right away and not use it than to need it and have to wait for it.

ALERT

AED

Do not use a cell phone or 2-way radio within 6 feet of an AED.

Determine the Need for an AED

As always, first check the victim's ABCs. If the victim is not breathing and has no signs of circulation, send someone to call 911 and to get an AED.

Start CPR

Remember BLS and the chain of survival. Give cardiopulmonary resuscitation (CPR) until the AED arrives at the scene and is ready to use. If you arrive at the victim with the AED, check the victim's ABCs and then use the AED immediately before starting CPR.

Attach the AED to the Victim

Be sure the victim is not in water or in contact with metal. Water or metal conduct electricity that may pose a risk to you or others. Place the AED near the victim's shoulder (on the left side if possible), turn it on, and attach the pads (electrodes) to the victim's chest.

Attach the AED pads to the victim only if the victim is unresponsive, not breathing and there are no signs of circulation (no movement, coughing, or breathing). Expose the victim's chest, and dry the skin with a towel or dry clothing (heart attack victims are often sweating). If the victim has heavy chest hair, quickly shave the pad areas. Remove the backing from the pads and apply the pads firmly on the victim's chest. If required with your AED model, plug the pad cables into the main unit.

Analyze and Shock

With the pads in place and the AED unit on, most AED models will automatically analyze the victim's heart rhythm. Do not move or touch the victim while it is analyzing. After it analyzes the heart rhythm the unit will advise you whether to give a shock. If a shock is advised be sure no one is touching the victim. Look up and down the victim and say, "Everybody clear!" Once everyone is clear administer the shock. After the shock the AED will analyze again and advise if another shock is needed. Up to three shocks are given in this way, and then the AED will advise you to check the victim and/or continue CPR. After 1 minute of CPR, the AED will repeat the whole process.

Note that different AEDs may use slightly different prompts. Follow the unit's words and picture prompts through this process. Many AEDs use a prompt that says "Check pulse" or something similar. As explained in Chapter 2, a pulse check should be performed only by those who have been trained to check for a pulse. Others should check instead for signs of circulation, which include breathing, coughing, movement, and normal skin condition.

If signs of circulation return after any shock, check the victim's breathing and continue to provide rescue breathing if necessary. Put an unresponsive, breathing victim in the recovery position and continue to monitor the ABCs. Keep the AED pads in place as some victims may return to V-fib and require defibrillation again.

The AED may also say no shock is indicated. This means the victim's heart will not benefit from defibrillation. If so, check the victim's ABCs again and give CPR if there are no signs of circulation.

Special AED Considerations

Some situations involve special considerations in the use of the AED.

AED Use in Children

Follow the adult guidelines for children over age 8. Although much more rare, sudden cardiac arrest can occur in younger children too from causes such as:

- Sudden infant death syndrome
- Poisoning
- Drowning

Perform the Skill

Using an AED

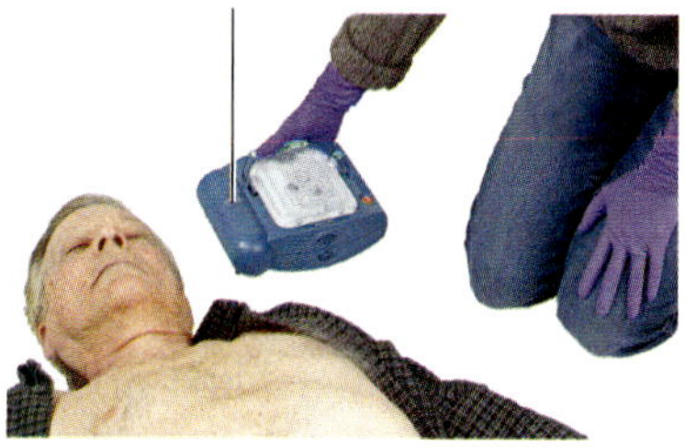

1 Position victim away from water and metal.

2 Place unit by victim's shoulder and turn it on.

3 Expose victim's chest, and dry or shave the area if necessary.

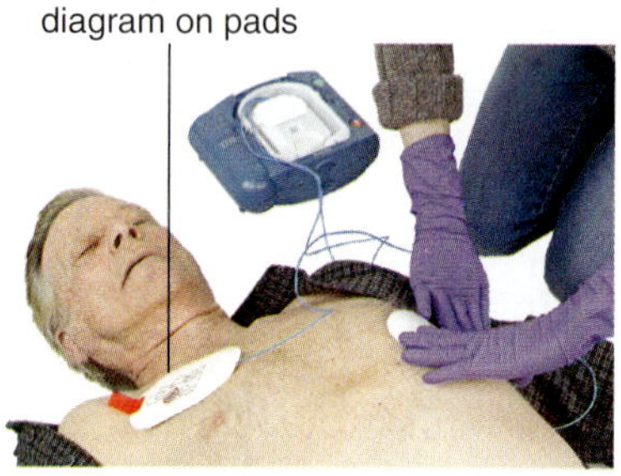

4 Apply pads to victim's chest. If needed, plug cables into unit.

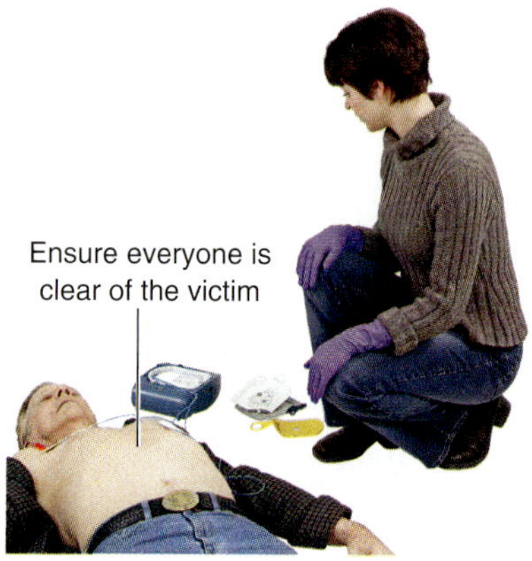

5 Stand clear during rhythm analysis.

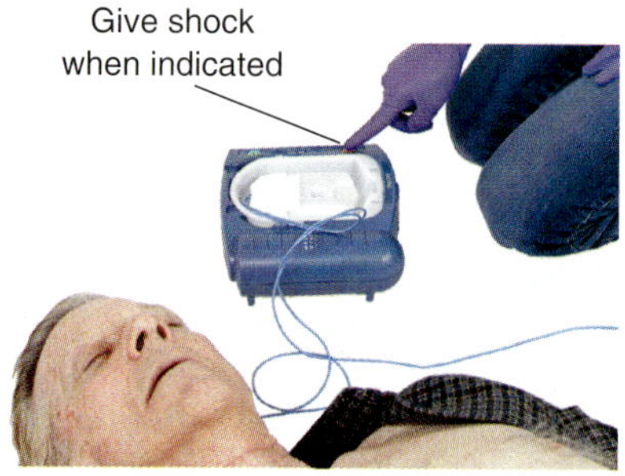

6 Follow prompts from AED unit to:
a. Press shock button or
b. Do not shock; check circulation, and give CPR if needed

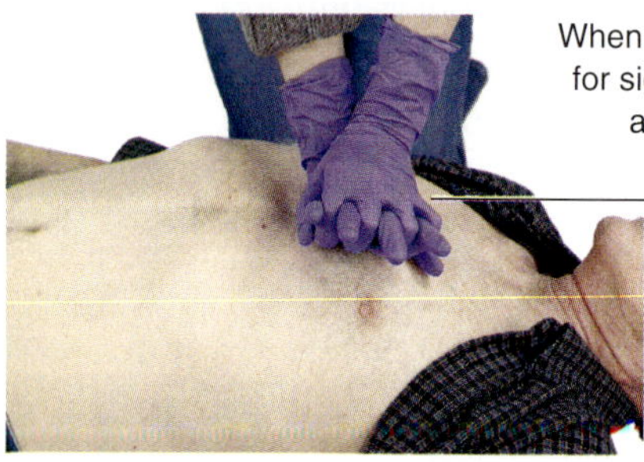

7 Follow prompts and your local protocol to administer sets of 3 shocks if needed, along with rechecking signs of circulation and giving CPR as needed.

8 If victim recovers, put in recovery position and monitor ABCs.

In recent years the value of defibrillating a young child in sudden cardiac arrest has been recognized, and pediatric AED electrode pads are now available. It is important to **use only approved pediatric AED electrode pads, which are smaller than those for adults and produce lower-energy shocks on a child under age 8. You should use an AED with pediatric electrode pads only if you have been trained with the equipment** (Figure 5-4).

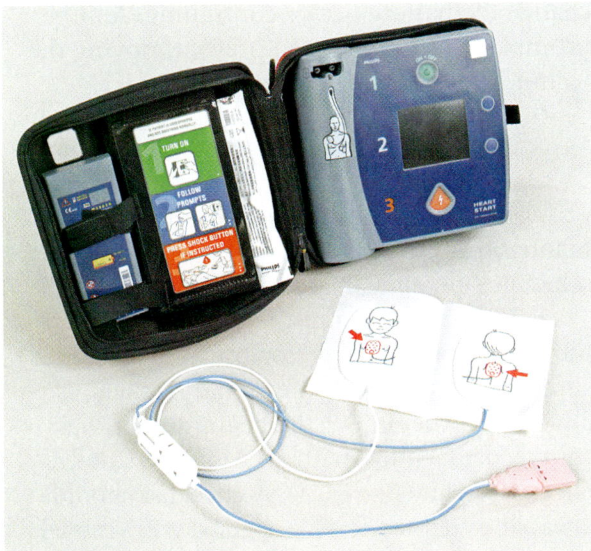

Figure 5-4 Pediatric AED unit.

Injured Victims

Cardiac arrest in a severely injured victim is usually caused by the traumatic injury, not by a heart rhythm problem like V-fib. In such cases your local medical direction may specify not to use the AED. However, if the injury seems minor, the victim's cardiac arrest may respond to defibrillation, and you should attach the pads and follow the prompts from the AED.

Victim with Internal Pacemaker or Defibrillator

When you expose the victim's chest to apply the AED pads, you may see a bulge beneath the victim's skin from an implanted pacemaker or defibrillator (**Figure 5-5**). Do not place a pad over this area but instead place it several inches away. If the victim's chest or body is jerking, there may be an implanted defibrillator that is giving shocks; wait until jerking has ended before applying the pads.

Hypothermia Victims

Determining signs of circulation in a victim of hypothermia (low body temperature) can be difficult. Handle a hypothermic victim very carefully because jarring may cause cardiac arrest. Follow your local guidelines for AED use if you find no signs of circulation. Typically, if the AED finds a shockable rhythm and advises shocks, only a total of three are given, and then CPR is performed until help arrives.

Victims with a Medication Patch

If the victim has a medication patch or paste on the chest, remove it and wipe the chest before applying the AED pads (**Figure 5-6**).

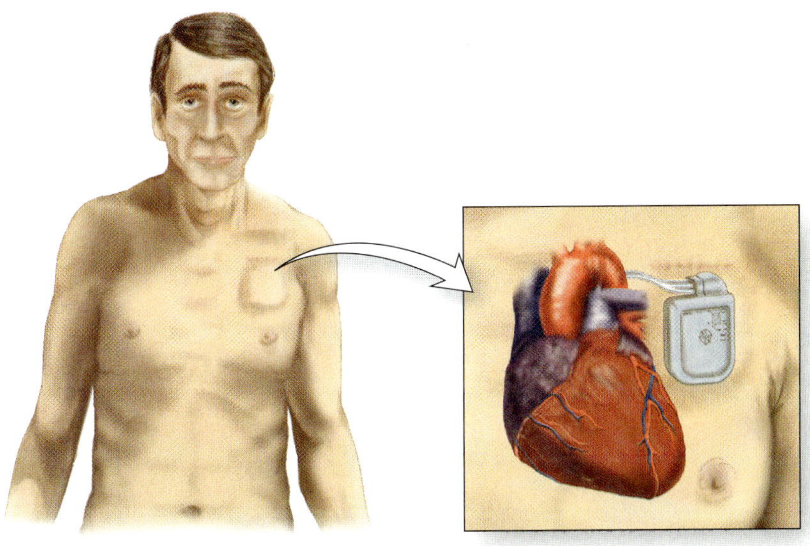

Figure 5-5 Vary AED placement if there is an internal device.

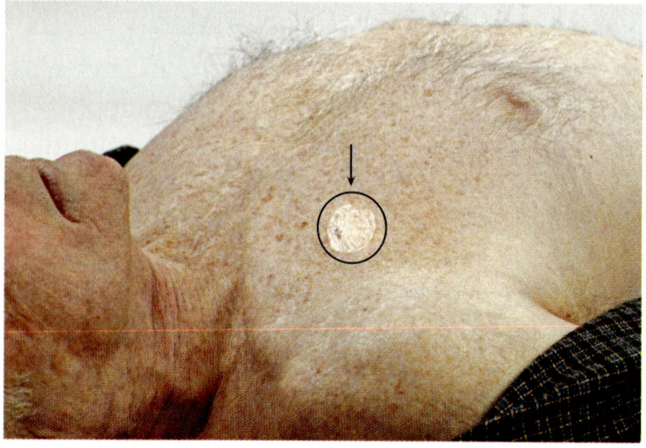

Figure 5-6 Remove medication patches prior to AED use.

Potential AED Problems

An AED must be maintained regularly and the battery kept charged. (See "AED Maintenance" section.) With regular maintenance an AED should not have any problems during use.

The AED may also prompt you to avoid problems. If you get a low battery prompt, change the battery before continuing. Another prompt may advise you to prevent moving the victim, if the AED detects motion.

AED Maintenance

AEDs require regular maintenance. Check the manual from the manufacturer for periodic scheduled maintenance and testing of the unit.

A daily inspection of the unit helps ensure the AED is always ready for use and all needed supplies are present. Professional rescuers usually inspect the unit at the beginning of their shift. Most facilities with an AED use a daily checklist form (**Figure 5-7**). A checklist should always be adapted for the specific AED model, including the manufacturer's daily maintenance guidelines. In addition, many units come with a simulator device to be used to check that the AED is correctly analyzing rhythms and delivering shocks; this may be part of the daily inspection routine.

A D

Date: ____________ Location: ________________ AED Model: ________________

Inspected by: ______________________ Signed: ________________________

AED unit		
verify correctly placed	____	____________
clean, clear of objects	____	____________
no cracks or damage to case	____	____________
cables/connectors present and not expired	____	____________
fully charged battery in place	____	____________
charged spare battery present	____	____________
check status/service light indicator	____	____________
check absence of service alarm	____	____________
power on, self-test	____	____________
Supplies	____	____________
Two sealed sets of electrode pads		
Verify expiration date on pad packages	____	____________
Razor	____	____________
Medical exam gloves	____	____________
Hand towels	____	____________
Alcohol wipes	____	____________
Scissors	____	____________
Pocket mask or face shield	____	____________

Figure 5-7 Example of an AED checklist.

Learning Checkpoint 1

1. True or False: An AED works by giving a shock to a heart that is fibrillating to restore it to a normal rhythm.

2. True or False: It is very risky to use an AED because the unit cannot tell whether the victim's heart is beating normally or not.

3. Which statement is true about the pads (electrodes) of an AED?

a. The AED has two pads which must be correctly positioned

b. The AED has four pads which must be correctly positioned

c. The AED has two pads, but only one needs to be put on the victim's chest (the other is a spare)

d. The pads are used only if a heart rhythm is not detected when the machine is placed in the center of the victim's chest

4. If the AED unit advises you to give a shock, what do you do next?

a. Continue CPR while asking someone else to push the shock button

b. Place a wet towel over the victim's chest and push the shock button

c. Make sure everyone is clear of the victim and then push the shock button

d. Do nothing except stay clear; the unit will automatically give the shock in about 10 seconds

5. An AED will usually advise giving a series of up to ____ shocks before advising you to stop and check for signs of circulation or give CPR.

6. Name at least one situation in which a young child may experience sudden cardiac arrest and could gain from use of a pediatric AED:

____

7. Describe where to put the AED pads if you see that a victim has an implanted pacemaker or defibrillator.

____

8. What should you do with the AED pads if the victim has a medication patch on the chest?

____

Appendix

A Summary of Basic Life Support

Step	Infant (under 1 year)	Child (1–8 years)	Adult (over 8 years)
1. Check for responsiveness	Stimulate to check response	"Are you okay" Tap shoulder	"Are you okay" Tap shoulder
2. If unresponsive, call 911	Send someone to call Give 1 minute of care before calling yourself if alone	Send someone to call Give 1 minute of care before calling yourself if alone (except for known heart problem)	Send someone to call Call immediately if alone (give 1 minute of care for victim of drowning, poisoning, injury)
3. If unresponsive: Open airway	Head tilt-chin lift (but do not overextend neck)	Head tilt-chin lift or jaw thrust	Head tilt-chin lift or jaw thrust
4. Check breathing	Look, listen, feel for breathing	Look, listen, feel for breathing	Look, listen, feel for breathing
5. If not breathing: Give 2 breaths, watch chest rise	Use barrier device or cover mouth/nose or nose Each breath lasts 1 to 1½ seconds	Use barrier device or cover mouth, or nose, or stoma Each breath lasts 1 to 1½ seconds	Use barrier device or cover mouth, nose, or stoma Each breath lasts 2 seconds
6. If chest does not rise Reposition airway and try 2 breaths again.	Each breath lasts 1 to 1½ seconds	Each breath lasts 1 to 1½ seconds	Each breath lasts 2 seconds

(continued)

Step	Infant (under 1 year)	Child (1–8 years)	Adult (over 8 years)
7. If chest still does not rise: Start CPR for airway obstruction (choking care)	For compressions use 2 fingers one finger-width below line between nipples Compress chest ½–1 inch Compress at rate of at least 100/minute 5 compressions per 1 breath	For compressions use one hand midway between nipples Compress chest 1–1½ inches Compress at rate of 100/minute 5 compressions per 1 breath	For compressions use both hands, one on top of other, midway between nipples Compress chest 1½–2 inches Compress at rate of 100/minute 15 compressions per 2 breaths
8. Check for signs of circulation	Scan body for movement, breathing, coughing, and normal skin condition	Scan body for movement, breathing, coughing, and normal skin condition	Scan body for movement, breathing, coughing, and normal skin condition
9. If circulation signs present but no breathing, give rescue breathing	1 breath every 3 seconds	1 breath every 3 seconds	1 breath every 5 seconds
10. If no signs of circulation present, continue CPR	Cycles of 5 compressions and 1 breath	Cycles of 5 compressions and 1 breath	Cycles of 15 compressions and 2 breaths
11. Continue to check for breathing and signs of circulation	Look, listen, and feel for breathing and scan body for signs of circulation	Look, listen, and feel for breathing and scan body for signs of circulation	Look, listen, and feel for breathing and scan body for signs of circulation
12. Use AED when available (if no breathing or signs of circulation)	Do not use AED	Use only pediatric electrode pads	Use adult AED electrode pads
13. If victim recovers breathing and signs of circulation, put in recovery position	Hold infant and monitor ABCs	Lay on side in recovery position and monitor ABCs	Lay on side in recovery position and monitor ABCs

Appendix

B Basic Life Support In Brief

Take Action in an Emergency

In Brief

1. Recognize the emergency.
2. Check the scene for safety.
3. Call 911 for life-threatening emergencies.
4. Assess the victim and provide first aid.

Assess the Victim

In Brief

1. Check the ABCs. Treat life-threatening conditions.
2. Get the victim's SAMPLE history.
3. Perform a physical examination.
4. Monitor victim for any changes in condition. For serious injuries recheck the ABCs at least every five minutes.

Rescue Breathing

In Brief

1. Open airway, and check victim's breathing.
2. If not breathing, position the barrier device.
3. Give 2 slow breaths, watching chest rise and fall.
4. Reposition to open airway, if needed, and repeat breaths.
5. Check for signs of circulation.
6. If signs of circulation are present, give one breath every 5 seconds (adult) or one breath every 3 seconds (child or infant).

Choking Adult or Child

In Brief

1. Encourage coughing if the victim is coughing and can breathe or speak.
2. Give abdominal thrusts if the victim indicates he or she cannot breathe or speak.
3. If victim becomes unresponsive, give CPR. Look in mouth for object before giving breaths in each cycle.

Choking Infant

In Brief

1. Give up to 5 back blows, look in mouth for object.
2. Give up to 5 chest thrusts, look in mouth for object.
3. Repeat back blows and chest thrusts.
4. If infant becomes unresponsive, give CPR. Look in mouth for object before giving breaths in each cycle.

CPR

In Brief

1. Open airway, and check victim's breathing.
2. Give 2 slow rescue breaths.
3. Determine if the victim has signs of circulation.
4. If no signs of circulation, start chest compressions.
5. Alternate chest compressions and rescue breaths (adult 15 to 2; child and infant 5 to 1).
6. Continue until victim has signs of circulation, an AED arrives, or someone else takes over.

Using an AED

In Brief

1. Use only when victim is not breathing and has no signs of circulation.
2. Place near victim's shoulder, turn on unit.
3. Apply pads to victim.
4. Follow AED unit prompts to analyze and give shocks.
5. Continue CPR if no shock advised and no signs of circulation.